TWO INCHES OF WOOL

The Simple Art of Self-Care

SUSAN L POKORNY

Dear Heidi,

I hope these pages bring you inspiration for rest, refreshment and renewal as you care for so many others. Multiply the Lord's goodness through your service! Thank you for your support and encouragement in this special project!

Blessings,
Sue
John 10:10

Contents

TWO INCHES OF WOOL

The Simple Art of Self-Care

Susan L. Pokorny
ERYT, TSHY

I dedicate this book to my family,
my sons and daughters.

To all sons and daughters,
may you find healing, wholeness and
purpose in your life.

To the many who work to care for the broken and the lost,
may you be lifted up and encouraged to keep pressing on.

Ackowledgements

Special Thanks and Acknowledgements

I have so many to thank for not only helping me finish this project, but everyone who has left an imprint on my life through care, mentoring, friendship, education and love.

To all those who've crossed my path in ministry, so many of you helped me flourish in friendship, leadership, and collaboration of so many opportunities. This project began years in my heart even before I knew it. It was formed and shaped by all of you as you modeled healthy relationships, mentoring and encouragement.

For my husband, Brad and each of my children who all endured months of my inspired creativity by listening, picking up extra chores and even helping edit excerpts of this manuscript and marketing materials. I've been blessed with a whole team of talent right in my own family. I love you all beyond words and feel so blessed that we are in this life together. You are all my inspiration for making a positive impact in this world and I pray this will bless you so you can be a light to those in your circles of influence.

To my parents, I would not be who I am today without the love and care you continue to show me even as an adult. Somewhere the world distracted me and I lost my way, but the seeds of faith, hope and love were always there waiting to be unearthed. The words thank you seem inadequate to package up a lifetime of love and devotion you continue to give. I hope I can follow in your footsteps of the love, respect and encouragement you show to everyone in your lives.

I'm grateful for the many counselors, teachers and clients in my life who have inspired me in this project as well as in healthy living for many years: Dr. Kim Anderson, Dr. Michelle Reyes, Dr. Frank & Sherry, Dr. Dennis, Krista Hull, Heidi Vance, Wendy Smith, Emmy, Holly, Kris, Karen, Rhonda, Lisa, Kim, KC, Cathy, Tresa and so many more. Thank you to Carrie Elliott Photography and Jenna Foscato of Tiffany Blue Photography. You are both amazing artists, compassionate and caring about the work you do reaching beyond the pictures and beautiful examples of authenticity and true confidence that you bring out in your clients.

Lastly, this project would not have been completed if it hadn't been for my dear friends. K. Paige Engle - my publisher and author coach, you kept me up when I was heading down, kept me on track and guided my every step to complete this. It would still be sitting in my computer files if I didn't have you by my side. You gave me the courage to step out and make this book a reality. Leah Stadel, my soul sister. Who would have known 17 years ago when our little boys were toddling together that one day we'd be working on this special project. As our families have grown, our hearts have come to see the same truths, hopes and potential for others. You have completed my thoughts on paper when I didn't realize they were there, organized a huge conglomeration of ideas into a living resource that will bless many. I love that you are a leader, mentor and speaker with LIFE Leadership and use your expertise and care as a former Music Therapist, RMT-BC. You truly have a gift with words, organization, insight and language that kept my content true to my spirit. You continue to brighten my life with the same positivity that has shined into the light of this book. Thank you.

Above all, I give all credit to the writing of this book to my Creator, the author of my life.

I pray this will be a blessing to many.

An Introduction

So, friend, how are you today?

What's going on in your life?

Are you feeling good?

What could be better?

From the moment we wake, in one way or another, we are tuning in to how we feel. There are questions you can ask yourself everyday. Is my physical body doing well or hurting a little? Am I excited to begin the day or do I dread getting out of bed? Is my soul downcast, lifted, or waiting to be stirred? We all feel something, but the degree to which we are aware of any or all of these feelings is the degree to which we are aware of our health. We wake each morning with a lifetime of experiences, habits, and idiosyncrasies from our past that shape our present awareness. This awareness is a sort of Wellness Quotient (WQ), something we can develop through decisions and directions that make up our life. If we make poor decisions physically, mentally, or emotionally, we become more disconnected or less whole. A soul is healthy and well-ordered when there is harmony between mind, body, and spirit. If we commit to habits that build up our health, mental and spiritual state, we can become more grounded and at peace. Being healthy isn't just about going to the gym, eating healthy foods or being educated or religious. Separately, these are all good practices, but when they are carried out with intention and awareness of their inter-connectedness, it takes our well-being to an entirely new level.

This inter-connectedness involves both self-awareness and a sense of wholeness. Self-awareness is similar to yet different from our sense of wholeness. Self-aware says I can tell there are parts and pieces of my life that are missing, broken or weak on one end of the spectrum, or vibrant, growing and strong on the other. A sense of wholeness says I can tell how my strengths and weaknesses are affecting each and every other area. It takes intentionality to bring about wholeness. If the enemy of self-awareness is distraction and avoidance, the enemy of wholeness is compartmentalizing. When we compartmentalize our lives, our focus can become fragmented. Wholeness of our mind, body, and spirit does not mean we live a life of perfection. When we begin to restore and reconnect with what makes each of us unique, with the goal of becoming more alive and present, we become more whole.

If the present is truly all we have, then tending to our health of body, mind and soul collectively allows for nurturing and healing from any past brokenness or future worry. There is a greater potential for balance as each piece begins to work as it was designed.

Each decision we make can be a form of worship when all the components of ourselves are working in unison towards the same goals of health, wellness, personal and spiritual growth. Harmony begins to establish a confidence in who we are, how unique we are, and orchestrates a life of continual growth and wellness. And this, my friend, is good for the soul.

So, friend, how are you today?

What's going on in your life?

Are you feeling good?

What could be better?

"May you realize that the shape of your soul is unique, that you have a special destiny here, that behind the facade of your life there is something beautiful, good, and eternal happening." [1]
-John O'Donohue

That's what this guide is all about, to show you that honest self-care leads to abundant living and tuned in senses so that you can be fully alive and present. Most likely you'll discover that when you create time for self-care, the choices you make will result in a few lost pounds, clearer thinking, more energy, and most importantly a deeper faith. This guide is the beginning of learning how to understand yourself better and equipping you to see yourself as a masterpiece. You need loving self-care to live in the fullness of your mind, body, and spirit. Have you ever thought of caring for yourself as an act of worship? Would you invite God into the tending of your mind, body, and your spirit? I promise you will never be disappointed in the decision to make Him your partner! Read on and take the next steps in discovering your God-intended potential on this two-inch piece of wool.

Chapter 1: Two Inches of Wool

The title for this book emerged from an email I received from one of my yoga students. "2 Inches of Wool" was the subject line. I had used this phrase a few times in the class earlier that week, and I hadn't realized the impact it had on my students until I received this note. The "two inches of wool" referred to a prop I use in most of my yoga classes. Each of my students begins class with a yoga mat and a wool blanket. The blanket is rather dense and unobtrusive, a boiled wool with simple gray fibers. It is folded to a sturdy, functional height of about two inches. I chose the blanket because wool is naturally water repellent, odor resistant and fairly sterile. It is also fire resistant. Practical. When the blanket is folded evenly, it offers a surprising softness that has stability and substance.

I offer students the option to sit on these two inches of wool at the beginning of class. They can use it throughout when they need a little bit more support under their body to shield it from a surface that might feel a bit too hard at the moment. I point out how this insulation may remind us of times we want to be shielded from difficult situations in our lives, or memories that are often painful to remember, even if only for an hour. Safe. I encourage them to try it and see if it makes a gentle difference as they enter into the presence of our class. Most students break into a surprised expression at the impact of this small prop. The wool also provides warmth and security: we can wrap ourselves in or softly cover ourselves if we feel cool or vulnerable during relaxation at the end of class. Comfort. Some days we feel the flames of adversity follow us onto our mat, but the wool blanket can extinguish the damaging heat at the moment. There is so much versatility, practicality and useful symbolism, and even spirituality in those two inches of wool.

My hope for this book is that it will bring together the earthly and spiritual considerations and practices of integrating our lives for whole health. The little routines or activities in this book are like the 2 inches of wool in my yoga class. On the surface, they might not seem like anything special, in fact many of them are just quite ordinary. But don't underestimate the power of each activity to have a big impact on our outlook, our physical health, or the fullness of our being. They will have significant effects not only in our life, but also the lives of those we interact with.

"The soul is the capacity to integrate all parts into a single, whole life. The soul seeks harmony, connection, and integration."

- Dallas Willard

Lost Sheep Found

I want you to know that this book was first written in my life story long before it was printed on these pages. What lies ahead in each chapter come from experience, education, revelation and constant reflection. To understand that better, let me share with you part of my story:

I woke most mornings weary when I should have been refreshed. I was constantly anxious, exhausted, dragging insomnia across my body. My mind was fogged with fear and depression. My small children woke full of energy but I was empty, an aching shell. By the age of 30, I already suffered pain in my hips and back, and my digestive track was a complicated mess. Physically, I was slowly manifesting the effects of too many processed foods, man-made chemicals and food sensitivities. I was emotionally unbalanced as a people-pleaser, frequently swinging others' needs far ahead of my own. Spiritually, I was searching for something, but despite being rooted in a church all my life, I had to admit I could not find bread or fruit that nourished my soul. In this season of chaos, I could not see a way to make my health and well-being a priority as I cared for a growing family. Adding to the story, I also worked outside of our home as a fitness instructor. My focus had mostly been on improving the physique of my body by any means whether it was losing the baby-fat or working to fit into my pre-pregnancy jeans. Nutrition, stress management, and non-toxic living were not part of the equation. Not enough? I was also expending any reserves I could muster up to volunteer my time and energy to good causes, most of which flowed to me, the people-pleaser, and pooled in my already surrendered swamp. Free movement and light-hearted play did not come easily. Bogged down and striving to meet everyone else's needs, I lost sight of who I was, what was important to me; I felt washed away and disconnected from how I was feeling physically and emotionally day-to-day. I had no idea that spiritually I was missing the biggest bridge, the deepest well. This was my life. This is what "living" was like for years.

Friend, we were originally designed to operate perfectly as physical, mental, emotional and spiritual beings. Our body's innate ability to develop and heal itself, our mind's capacity to conceive, adapt, reframe, and expand ideas, our ability to feel and respond emotionally, and our innate sense of longing spiritually are all signs that we were created by someone for something. We are each living at less than 100% capacity and any given moment, some of us are teetering on brokenness, as I was. Others are climbing higher and seeing farther with each step. We sense we can be more, do more, and give more. We each desire to find satisfaction and peace in achieving our potential, to become more and more who we were intended to be in every way. To be **self-aware** and full of life, this is living. This is something I longed for, and perhaps you do, too.

"All of us have moments like this, glimpses of our true creation. They come unexpectedly and then fade again. Life for the most part keeps our glory hidden, cloaked by sin, sorrow, or merely weariness."
- John Elderidge

As a former competitive gymnast, I knew what it was to be **self-aware**. I experienced the discipline of mental and physical strength that came from endless hours of skillful practice and focus. These skills are universally adaptable for growth in any area, but because of their intensity, we often do not continually apply them in all we do. And with time, discipline like any other muscle can erode. Often it takes a crisis or a great need to remind us of these powerful practices. As I was struggling those early years of motherhood, I slipped further away from the self-awareness of a gymnast into a free fall of self-forgetfulness as mother/wife/friend/employee/volunteer. But the proverbial crisis did come, and it was a real turning point of my self-care. With one horrific moment, I was thrust into a journey of awakening. I don't advocate waiting for a crisis situation before embracing self-care. Hopefully you'll be able to apply these principles before the storms come. Then you will be able to meet those challenges with a better outlook and foundation of well-being.

The thing about crisis is that it's often unexpected. I was six months pregnant with our daughter and had two boys under the age of three. My husband, Brad, was in the backyard burning leaves when the flames caught hold of him, and within seconds, he was burned over 50% of his body. These were third degree burns mostly, which destroyed the outer layer of his skin and the entire layer beneath. During the following three months of hospitalization, he endured countless surgeries and a battle for his life as I stood by his side praying, supporting and doing all I could to encourage him.

During these three months, God made it clear to me that we were not going to walk this path alone. This was my first awareness. I felt an unspeakable yet undeniable sense of His grace and love washing over me, bringing peace and understanding. He was with us every moment in a way I had never experienced before. My spirit instinctively rose to meet this peace and continually received it freely to get through what lay ahead.

Just as important as my spirit and faith being re-awakened, I became aware of the great circle of family and friends that surrounded me. There were many who came to pray with us, bring us meals, help us care for our little ones and shower us with care. During this time of healing, our friends and family gave us much needed support, which we received with gratitude as one does with a lifeline when drowning at sea.

There are many days I look back and realize how God used each person in our lives in that season. I was even protected physically, as I carried our baby girl on to full term in a healthy delivery. Brad arrived home one week before our beautiful daughter was born, a testimony of faithfulness and hope of better things to come.

Emotionally we never had to carry Brad's burden alone. We were supported spiritually through countless prayers that God answered through His comfort, peace and provision. Through all these acts of kindness, I was transformed in my understanding that I needed care and was worthy of receiving care from others. It happened so completely that I revolutionized my thinking and I internalized how important it was for me to care for myself and my unborn daughter. We experienced so much assistance in practical matters, but I also grew a deeper appreciation for the little blessings in my life: being able to see my children laugh and play, seeing the sun come out after a week of snowy, cloudy weather, and the kind words of a stranger. These were everyday blessings that I could be thankful for and receive with a new open heart. Everything broken that needed recreating in our life healed as Brad healed. We not only survived, we truly learned how to live again.

"God has given us two hands, one to give, the other to receive"
- Billy Graham

After my husband had recovered and we once again took hold of the wheel of our family, things were different. Having experienced the gift of being ministered to and cared for by others for three long months, I knew the full value of self-care. I felt compelled to take more responsibility for my care, and because of all we had gone through, I could do it at a deeper level. The sense of love we experienced wrapped around us and that caring changed me. It wasn't superficial by any measure. My focus on healthy eating and removing chemicals from our household happened because I took ownership of my thoughts and actions. I wasn't simply making choices because others said I should do so, but because I sensed this was the right path to wholeness in my mind, body and spirit. This new season of self-care was the beginning of spiritual acts of worship in response to God's faithfulness and love; I wanted to honor God, my creator and sustainer by tending to everything He created me to be. This is where I began seeing the deep connection between mind, body and spirit.

Faith-based exercise was an integral tool to bringing me back to my creator, to my senses, helping me find balance, better self-awareness and confidence in my physical being. My fitness training was the place I discovered a divine sense of why I should treat my body as a temple of the Holy Spirit. For Christians, it is not only in the mind or heart that God dwells, but also our bodies, making each cell, bone, muscle and organ a sacred space. Caring for my body as a temple of the living God is the ultimate way I can honor this gift of life He has given me. Working with the Holy Spirit in this discipline of worship does not mean that I have a perfect body without pain or sickness, but it does encourage the calm and hopeful faith that my life is in His hands. And as our earthly bodies are temporary, but the mind and spirit eternal, I began to live in the fullness of who I am in Christ: mind, body and spirit woven together in an elaborate holy tapestry.

"Don't you know that you yourselves are God's temple and God's Spirit dwells in your midst? God's temple is sacred and you together are that temple."
1 Corinthians 3:16-17, New International Version

In the years following that divine crisis, the Pokorny lives continued on in a good direction. We are far from perfect, but have gained a dynamic faith, a steady growth and deepening of friendships, and a more holistic view of our health and well-being. What about you and your family? Are you one of the millions in our culture, like we were, not managing stress well, living in survival mode, or lacking abundance? Have you lost sight of who you really are and who you are created to be? Do you live out an existence where balance, restoration, or calm seems unimaginable? It is an interesting thing that often others around us may see the gaps in our care where we have become numb or oblivious. Often the biggest obstacle we have is giving ourselves permission to pause, assess our life, and begin to do a better job in any or all of these areas. But it is in my heart to tell you, there is hope! You can live with peace, satisfaction, and confidence no matter what your circumstances are.

"What is it that your heart needs? Peace? Satisfaction? Wholeness? I can bring into being that which doesn't currently exist if you'll just soak in My words. Not only will they wash away the hurt of your past, but they will also illuminate your future. Are you wondering what your next steps should be? I'll tell you if you let Me wash you in My word. Be careful not to just listen to the words, but act on them. If you do, you'll find that the comfort I pour into your heart will be more than enough to heal you - enough to be shared with other broken people." [2]
-Dannah Gresh

Chapter 2: What You Can Find Here

Who This Book Is For

There are a lot of self-help books on the market with some great information, and I hope you are always curious to learn more. But this book is especially dedicated to those among us who have experienced struggles or a trauma that have fractured the mind-body-spirit connection. If your soul is hurting or carrying past trauma or emotional baggage it may eventually lead to physical illness - if it hasn't already, and likely pervades your thinking in subtle or not-so-subtle ways. You will find that learning and applying increasingly good self-care habits such as eating whole foods, exercising, getting sufficient sleep and water are a few examples that can be game changers in your well-being and your spiritual walk. You may also find that in tending to your soul and finding an increasing peace will lead your physical and mental state to become stronger. You have survived many things and along the way may have come to rely on some habits that have distracted or comforted you; but perhaps some of these habits have kept you from the wholeness you long to feel. You want to change, but because none of us instinctively knows what practices can help, you might be a little lost in where to start.

Well, you're here! And that's a great start for which you need to be congratulated! Just taking responsibility to begin is a step in the right direction. This guide is specifically designed in a simple to use format with the basics of wellness, nutrition, physical movement and mind-body exercises to bring it all together one step at a time. It was intentionally made to give you options to explore a new practice, to reconsider some old thoughts, and to explore connecting with a loving God, all which bring about health and wellness for your soul.

"As a culture, we have outsourced many roles and much of the wisdom that used to be primarily present and taught in the home. What was once passed on from parent to child is now an industry. Here are just some of the primary examples of what we now pay others to teach or do for us:

· Childcare

· Education

· Eldercare

· Counseling

· Food Production/Cooking

· Home Repair

· Cleaning

· Massage Therapy

· Entertainment

· Sexual Intimacy

· Animal Care

· Yard/Property Care

· Role Modeling

· Teaching Religion/Faith"

- OLIVER DEMILLE [3]

This list can really cause us to stop and ask ourselves some questions. How much do I really know about my own health? How did I learn what I do know? How much more can I learn? It is quite amazing what goes into daily living and affects our health. Of all these topics and practices, however, Two Inches of Wool is dedicated more to educating ourselves on proper thinking and habits, food and environment choices, and how to grow our awareness of the relationship between our mind, body, and spirit. You may have heard the saying 'we don't know what we don't know'. That's ok, none of us will ever know everything. This book will be a place you can safely discover what you don't know. There is no judgement of where you are in the journey, just encouragement of moving forward to a better place, physically, emotionally, spiritually. If you haven't been shown these routines in a caring, loving place, you can find it here.

What Is Self-Care?

Beauty is in the eye of the beholder, or so it is said. Art has an element of subjectiveness, an aspect of the unknown, where often the process is just as important as the finished project. In art, all components are important: the foundation of the piece (the canvas), the tools that are used (brushes, paints) and the completed work of art. Two artists can begin a project with the exact same materials and create a completely different piece.

This is art: the same tools, different perspectives and a unique piece of art.

Likewise, Self-care is also an art because there is not one specific answer or path for every single person. Our beliefs are the foundation of our artwork that will guide our direction, our tools are the choices we make each day to nourish our physical body, emotions, attitudes and our spiritual selves. The masterpiece we are becoming is how our spirit engages with others in our community and in our faith.

All societies have values of how each individual fits into the place of communities. Our modern culture places a great emphasis on self-improvement, self-promotion and success based on taking charge of our own destiny in personal and professional growth. While these actions are not bad in and of themselves as it's important for us to be assertive and responsible for our own lives, they are for the most part focused on the exterior. Self-promotion runs the risk of losing a sense of "others" that is integral in genuinely connecting with those around us.

Self-care on the other hand, is guided by the interior. We may care for the exterior, the physical body, in some ways such as through good nutrition, but it's the care of our emotional selves that is the starting point to connecting with others outside of ourself. Self-care is driven by the fullest sense of who we are and our need to be whole: caring for our physical body with reasonable diet, exercise and rest, nurturing our emotional selves by building healthy relationships driven by pure motives, and feeding our spirit with grounded faith.

Caring for our self goes beyond health and nutrition and gives us a sense of what we need, when we need it. If we are in a stressful situation or working overtime in any area of our life, stepping into Self-Care gives us the place to pause, reflect and manage our emotional and spiritual selves as well as caring for our physical body. This is the place we step into unison of all our working parts to bring them in harmony with one another: mind, body and spirit. When we can manage ourselves in this holistic care, it gives us a stronger foundation to care for others. Anyone working in high-stress occupations run the risk of burnout or breakdown so self-care is essential to continuing meaningful work that is life-giving for the care-giver and the receiver.

All of these parts working in unison towards the same goals is where we discover real wholeness. If one part is lacking or moving in another direction, the other areas will suffer and we experience a disconnect in ourselves. For example, if you are strong in your faith and eating a balanced diet but you carry trauma from years ago this can affect your physical body and possibly create strongholds in your life. Maybe you're emotionally strong and committed in your faith but are not treating your body as a temple in the way you care for your physical body. Eventually, neglecting the physical body will impact other areas of your body, even your brain health which could raise the risk off suffering from anxiety, depression or other disease. Every area of our life needs tending to in a loving way, you deserve that!

"Two Inches of Wool" is dedicated to paving the pathway to holistic wellness for your mind, body and spirit, to help you discover how to live a life of wholeness - even in the midst of a storm. Self-care builds up the framework of who you are so you don't get tossed about in the ocean of uncertainty, you are anchored in the hope of who you are and who you were created to be. Authentic self-care honors who you are. As you discover a better sense of yourself, the choices you make in mind, body and spirit will become easier and more clear.

Self-care is an art, just like we have the art of conversation. When we interact with other people, we cannot define all the rules of what to say and what not to say in any given circumstance. For example, if you meet someone at the airport and begin to talk with them about their trip your responses will vary based on the information they give you. If your conversation focuses on the latest news or insight to a business trip, your verbal cues will adjust to fit the situation. Maybe they are taking a trip with young children so your conversation may include the little ones. The art of Self-care is no different. There are some tried and true "rules" of self-care that involve good nutrition, exercising regularly, healthy relationships and tending to our spiritual self, but it also involves many nuances like the art of conversation. If you are a single, working professional who travels a lot, the choices you make may look different than if you are a married, work at home mom with several children.

The principles of how to care for yourself don't change - the essence of which is treating your body as a sacred temple of the Holy Spirit: caring for your mind, body and spirit. How we each carry out the principles may look different in each of our lives. This is the foundation of our artwork, the core of Self-care: discovering what will work in your life right now so you can continue to grow in knowledge of yourself and make the best choices you can to discover wholeness, wellness and peace where you are. Are you ready to jump in and begin creating your piece of art? Let's get started!

Visiting A New Culture

I want to take a moment here for those of you who struggle with the faith and spiritual dimension of your life. I realize for many of us, there is a tangle and confusion as to how religion, faith tradition and spirituality add to our sense of wholeness. And let me assure you, the many questions that arise in this area are ones all of us confront at one time or another. I would simply encourage you to try two things if this is your area of struggle: find someone you respect and trust who has a stronger faith and ask them to share the resources they use so you can move in that same direction. Secondly, keep an open mind as you read with me. I can't speak about many of the ways people seek spiritual peace, I can only speak from what I know. The results I have come from following a Christian tradition, specifi-cally a personal relationship with Jesus Christ. You won't find me pointing to a religion or a denomination, but you will find me explaining what Christ has shown me through his Word (the Bible) in connecting mind, body and spirit in my life. If you don't share this faith, I encourage you to keep an open mind, just as if you were visiting another culture. Perhaps you might just simply consider that the Bible is one of the oldest historical documents in the world and is filled with encouraging words that heal. You'll find many biblical verses within these chapters that can be powerful in shaping the framework of your thoughts.

"Discovery comes not in seeking new lands,
but in seeing with new eyes."
- Marcel Proust

Change is not always easy, but we often experience the most growth when we move through the uncomfortable. This is the place that you can face the unknown with courage and gentleness as you discover the real treasures in your life and experience the rewards of insight, understanding and peace.

What This Book Is Not

Nothing is more ignored than complicated theoretical "how-to" books, lists or ideas. Even complicated recipes remain just photos untasted. Ingredients you can't find, items you can't pronounce or techniques that require ongoing support from experts online or in a studio are merely roadblocks to someone who seeks a believable and simple path. Therefore, you won't find any of that here. Having said that, please keep in mind that this book also isn't a substitute for medical care or counseling that you may come to recognize you want or need. Rather, it is a tool you can use independently or with a counselor to compliment any types of therapies. This guide will help you make the most of your natural instincts, your intuition and need for self-care. The principles and suggestions within these pages have been collected, shared, practiced by holistic practitioners and everyday people who just want to live a cleaner, more authentic life that supports natural living, pure self-care and wholeness in their mind, body, and spirit.

"Tell me and I'll forget, Teach me and I'll remember, Involve me and I'll learn."
- Ben Franklin

How To Use This Book

This book has been designed as a quick reference to ebb and flow with your life. It is divided into three distinct areas with specific useful strategies and considerations in each.

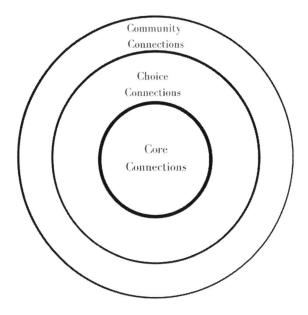

Connections

As I mentioned in the opening of this book, our goal is to live out a more connected life between our mind, body and spirit. Each of these main sections will focus on the resources and thought patterns that can influence how interconnected these areas will be. The path you take to connecting these parts will be very personal and happen in a more organic way as you apply principles and prompts to your own life and personal situation.

1. A CORE CONNECTION: These are practices that address **foundational thinking** in understanding yourself.

2. A CHOICE CONNECTION: These are practices that address **lifestyle choices** which take us closer to or farther from healing and wholeness.

3. A COMMUNITY CONNECTION: These are practices that **continue and extend beyond ourselves** and provide a healing in our ability to connect and impact the community around us. These activities help develop our sense of purpose, value and intentional living with others.

So, my friend, let's begin!

CORE CONNECTIONS

Foundational Thinking
and
Understanding Yourself

Chapter 3: Building Self-Awareness

THE STARTING AND ENDING POINT OF HEALTH

"Your soul is what integrates your will (your intentions), your mind (your thoughts and feelings, your values and conscience), and your body (your face, body language, and actions) into a single life. A soul is healthy - well-ordered - when there is harmony between these three entities and God's intent for all creation. When you are connected with God and other people in life, you have a healthy soul." [4]

- John Ortberg, Soul Keeping

Self-Awareness Defined

Self-awareness is the observation of how well the mind, body and spirit are working together. The feedback and insights gained by meditation or prayer and through interactions with others can provide better insight into how healthy we are. There are likely some areas in your life where you have a high degree of awareness, but equally, there may be some areas that need to be explored. The encouraging news here is that there are daily habits that can help you "tune in" and explore. For example, practicing daily mediation and prayer allows the mind and spirit to:

25

- Step away from busy-ness and noise.
- Create a space for your mind to review significant situations and activities you are experiencing.
- Allow your spirit to reveal feelings and intuitions you are having about those experiences.
- Take an opportunity to make new decisions about your perspectives of them.

Meditation can be a loosely defined practice depending on what source you seek. In Two Inches Of Wool, meditation refers to a form of deep thinking that comes from the Hebrew word Sihach which means to muse, contemplate or diligently consider [5] as in the Biblical verses of Psalm 119. Many modern forms of meditation might teach to empty the mind or listen to guided meditations with a teacher's lead. When the term "meditate" is used in this book, I encourage you to use an active approach to holding your thoughts captive, consider them and acknowledge them in the present moments as defined by this Hebrew word Sihach.

In a Psalm of David, "May the words of my mouth and the meditations of my heart be pleasing in your sight" [6] In this sense, what thoughts do you surround yourself with? When you meditate and hold your thoughts captive, you will most likely be faced with thoughts that you've had in the past that do not align with who you want to be. Meditation can be an opportunity to "re-train" your brain into positive thinking and awareness of your thoughts and actions day to day. Practicing this type of "meditation" is a form of mindfulness to bring intention to your thoughts.

Another way to think of this quiet, thoughtful meditation is to consider the Hebrew word "hahah". Hagah also means to meditate, but in a sense of how words may enter our soul, just as food enters our body in an active way. Chewing and swallowing, using teeth and tongue, tasting and savoring, anticipating and taking in the sweet and spicy, mouth-watering and soul-energizing morsel words.[7] When we meditate on thoughts and words in this way it nourishes us by becoming fully absorbed into who we are, just as the blood flows and permeates every cell in our body. This intention can help form deeper thoughts and insight that reaches every part of your life.

It can be extremely difficult to track patterns in your thinking, your emotions, and honestly, your stress levels without regular meditation and prayer thoughts. Without attending to your life in this manner, it is as though the car is driving down the road but there is no driver! Can you imagine driving down a (life's) highway and seeing car after car moving along completely unattended? You would certainly expect some major crashes to happen and many other cars wandering into ditches, completely off the road, off purpose.

Practicing self-awareness is truly a life-long skill development, but the rewards are enormous. There may be times when it is difficult to determine what is off either physically, mentally or emotionally. It may be that more time and frequent revisiting are needed. It may be that new information, new learning reveals something about yourself you simply didn't know before. When there is an area we lack awareness in, we can go so far as to say we are "self-deceived". For example, if I come back from a check-up from my doctor and find my blood pressure is great, my cholesterol is great and I have no aches, pains or diseases, I could consider myself a pretty healthy person. But if in the lobby I meet a friend who works out several times a week, practices healthy eating habits, and manages her time well, all the while knowing I don't do any of that, am I truly that healthy? No, I am self-deceived because in due time, those unattended areas will be just like that unattended car, and I will crash. So taking time to learn new things about what keeps me healthy is a big part of being self-aware.

An additional benefit to practicing self-awareness is building strength to change old destructive habits. By taking time to meditate or pray, you buy space to react to situations and events, which almost always leads to better responses. Reactive people only deal with situations as they arise, often from a more emotional-centered perspective. When we're pro-active we take time to consider and ponder before we react. When we pause we have time to respond with intention and care from what we've just observed. Even physical awareness works this way: having chronic pain and not taking time to assess how it is affecting our mind and spirit can lead to feelings of helplessness and depression. By practicing self-awareness, new attitudes and decisions about how to manage the pain physically, emotionally, mentally and spiritually can go a long way in protecting our quality of life.

Self-awareness will eventually lead to self-acceptance, but it will also lead to deeper healing.

THE ABILITY TO take control of your life and feel empowered directly affects your happiness and well-being. This is not anything one person can do for another; this is very personal and private work. It is the essence of being mindful and intentional, vigilant and self-aware. Once you know yourself better, it is easier to see others more honestly and accept them for who they are as well. This creates a greater peace within ourselves that extends to the people around us.

Cultivating Self-Awareness

Developing self-awareness takes time and dedication. It's an ongoing process and there is no end-point, but there is a growing satisfaction that comes with understanding ourselves at a deeper level. We can begin to build awareness when we try and understand what outside influences might be directing our actions, our priorities and beliefs.

To begin, I would recommend you write out a timeline of your life which includes key events and memories. This will take time and patience, but you can begin slowly by writing your earliest memories in a simple notebook. Include anything significant - good or bad - that comes to mind. Make sure to include any significant injuries to your physical body, strong emotional events or spiritual markers.

Leave space between events to fill in any thoughts, emotions or other memories that might be a part of those initial notes.

There is no right or wrong way to do this; the importance of it is to reflect on those earlier experiences and see how they may have shaped you into the person you are today. As you progress, continue to add any new information that you might remember or reflect on to add to your self-awareness. This simple record of your "story" can be a great beginning to understanding yourself better.

Instead of running from your past, face it with courage. Accepting your past doesn't mean you grieve the brokenness any less. Grieving is a areal part of the healing process. Honoring this natural process is where real insight and awareness occur.

Following each writing session, take time to reflect on them as the adult you are today. Identify things that:

· May still be a struggle

· Could use a new perspective

· Have formed a stronger character in you (good things and bad)

· You are grateful for

· Things you want to improve

Mindfulness and vigilance can follow better when you have more self-awareness of your physical body, emotions and spiritual self. Vigilance is keeping watch over the choices you make and the relationships you develop to keep or bring them into alignment with your core values and the unity of your mind, body and spirit.

And the opposite of vigilance is distraction…

The Dysfunction of Distraction

DISTRACTION

dis 'trac' tion

1. Confusion of affairs; disorder; detachment.

2. A drawing apart; separation.

3. Dividing attention. Prevents concentration.

The Information Age has become the Distracted Era. As our culture develops great technologies to manage information, business operations and maximize automation, it's even more important to hold onto developing the skills that rest on our humanity. Our humanness is what relates to another person in genuine connection, eye contact, physical touch, chemistry and emotional understanding when we are in person. The five senses remind us we are active and living.

Technology breeds distraction.

Heads down, checking emails in the middle of dinner conversations has socially become the norm. Relational distractions. Performance standards have moved beyond weight in the search for anti-aging, memory-enhancing, disease-curing answers. Physical distractions. Endless searching for questions and answers, social media monitoring, information retrieval; more data than we can absorb in a lifetime. Emotional and spiritual distractions.

How do we manage? Pushing our minds, bodies and spirits to the limit. Physically, we can fuel our low energy reserves by artificial means. Our active minds and busy schedules can become an obstacle to deep thinking and forming long-lasting relationships. Spiritually, we have a smorgasbord of thoughts and ideas to choose from. How do we manage all these distractions? The simple answer is artificially.

The Western world has the mood and energy-enhancement industries making trillions of dollars. According to the Center for Disease Control, 9 million Americans use prescription sleep aids to fall asleep. The study concluded, "most are white, female, educated and 50 or older…" But that's only part of the picture. Experts believe there are millions more who try options like over-the-counter medicines or chamomile tea, or simply suffer through sleepless nights."[8] By day, Americans trying to stay awake are consuming 400 million cups of coffee from restaurants, coffee houses and gas stations. Millions more are brewing pots at home.[9] Our mid-day energy-crisis is solved by purchasing $8.1 billion of energy drinks and shots.[10][11] I was one of these statistics in the years after I graduated from college. My 70-hour work week was fueled by my intake of coffee, diet soda and yogurt.

Feeling down? Spray some mountain sunshine in the air (in the form of chemical fragrance) to the tune of 357 million purchases a year.[12] What are we seeking in this overstimulated, chemical-saturated society? An alert, happy demeanor? A sharper mind? A sense of peace? Thicker hair? Brighter skin? Slimmer waist? Acceptance? Self-esteem? Shelter from guilt? Happiness? Contentment? Avoidance of tough issues? Relief of discomfort in any form?

The answers won't be found in any product, at least not long term. You may be happy for a short time, but the moment will fade.

The heart of distraction is our self. If we are tuned out of ourselves, distracted, we lose perspectives of how our external choices are really affecting us physically, emotionally, spiritually. If we cannot gauge what we are really feeling physically, emotionally, spiritually, how can we truly determine the "who", "what", "when", "how", "why" of any situation and make concise, focused decisions? When we are tuned out of our self, distraction is more likely to happen.

What if the answers were found right within us? Have you ever considered that the more you become aware of your senses, the less you will seek satisfaction in material things, food or dysfunctional relationships? I was stuck in that endless search many times myself without realizing it. I was shifting from one place and website to the next, looking for answers to what were probably wrong questions. I didn't have a compass, a direction or purpose to guide me. I wandered aimlessly, picking up a good habit here, or a few healthy eating tips there, but seldom did anything stick. Because I didn't have a confident understanding of myself, I allowed advertising, main stream media and other influences to leave me wandering in the desert with no distinct end point or reason to it all other than a slimmer waistline and a mood-enhanced smile. The problem was there was always a new antioxidant, a new product or diet that might offer a solution to what I was searching for at the moment. Entire industries were up and running ready to give me a search-engine answer; the ease of typing a question and receiving a well-marketed answer became a habit, all the while I was missing the big picture. Our bodies are not a combination of individual operating systems functioning on their own where a single question and single answer will suffice. We are complex beings. Every cell in our body is interconnected. Scientists have made amazing discoveries about the human mind and body, but there are still many aspects known only by our creator including how we are all connected with each other and all of creation. What we seek is integration, not product application. When we are focused and tuned into our self, we can better see how individual choices we make every day will impact us physically, emotionally, spiritually as a whole rather than dealing with a simple question-answer pattern that technology delivers.

Wrong question + answer = Distraction

This is your life and you are the only one who can take responsibility for it. It's not as complicated as some would make it seem. Part of your design is the ability to assess yourself and sense a problem. Finding an integrated approach to solve your problem happens when you identify it and take note of how it is affecting you physically, mentally, emotionally and spiritually. It really is as systematic as that. For example, if you are constantly tired, ask yourself:

1. How is my body resting?
2. How is my mind or thinking contributing to restlessness?
3. What emotions are present when I am tired?
4. What does my spirit long for in this deprivation?

"If you take responsibility for anything in your life, know that you'll feel fear. That fear will manifest itself in many ways: fear of embarrassment, fear of failure, fear of hurt. Such fears are entirely natural and healthy, and you should recognize them as proof that you've chosen work worth doing. Every worthy challenge will inspire some fear." [13] -Eric Greatness

One of the most important steps you can take in adopting these principles into your life is to begin to detox from marketing. Advertisers tell us how we should feel, building a facade of confidence in what we consume or whom we follow. We want to be confident with the choices we make, we want studies to prove those choices are right and we want experts to confirm that we are doing the best we can. We want to follow our friends. The problem arises when one expert contradicts another, or our body doesn't respond the way the research predicted or we follow paths that take us to places that are just a distraction. Confusion sets in, allergic reactions arise, side effects emerge and distract us from our original problem, complicating the matter. After time, doubt creeps in. When we expect our well-being to rest on a packaged product we use, shaped by the brands we wear and the stuff we buy, we cause a disconnect between our true selves and how we perceive we should be living. When we have a reaction to a supposedly safe prescription drug from an educated doctor, we question our intuition or gut instincts.

Throughout my self-care revolution, I've experienced plenty of distractions which resulted in confusion. As I practiced self-awareness and began to understand my responses to outside stimuli, I gained a clearer understanding of how my physical body and emotions were affected by many circumstances. Surprisingly, this insight became apparent during the delivery of one my children.

When I gave birth to our 6th child, I was in the same hospital as I had been for the previous five births. I had a couple of challenging deliveries, but the previous 2 had gone pretty smoothly so I had a good outlook for what lay ahead. I had planned a natural birth, but as the due date came and went with no labor pains in sight, I was given a pitocin induction. Because no guarantees were given as to how long the induction would take, I was also prescribed a walking epidural. When the anesthesiologist arrived, I mentioned I had had an allergic reaction to something in the narcotic cocktail administered during my first delivery, and that subsequent doctors were able to avoid that medication in the next few. That instigated a search through my past records, which a nurse informed me would take six hours as they were currently transferring documents to electronic form. The doctor decided he did not want to wait that long, and proceeded to administer the meds. Within minutes I knew something was wrong; I felt my blood pressure dropping and my limbs going numb. In a panic, I called for the nurse telling her what I observed. Within 30 minutes she was back with my paper files (much quicker than six hours) and said she saw the notes indicating my allergy. She disconnected the narcotic with not so much as an apology. I was not a happy camper and needless to say, I now carry a list of my medication allergies with me at all times. My assertiveness at the time didn't come easy as I felt intimidated talking with a well-educated doctor and nurse, but I'm thankful I had the body awareness to know something wasn't right. You have that awareness as well; it may be hidden underneath insecurity or past trauma, but you can find it again and become stronger. You can learn to understand yourself better than many professionals; in fact, there are even some professionals who know that your personal awareness is KEY in their treatment for you.

Before going on, I want to acknowledge that sometimes we have a tendency to look back at choices we've made and feel guilty for not knowing better. While it's important to have some amount of reflection in our lives to observe choices we've made, it is much more important to use it to grow stronger and motivate yourself to make new choices. Extending personal grace in the process of discovery will help us master the tools we're learning to use.

Removing distractions can build margins into our day to focus on what really matters in our life.

When we remove distractions we can build in margins to focus on what really matters in our life. When you give yourself space for reflection, clearer thinking often follows. I want you to enjoy this journey of discovery and never feel guilty for the past.

"The truth is, we all fall down. We all mess up and make mistakes and do and say the wrong things sometimes. But the beauty is in the recovery. It's in the way you handle yourself as you pick up the pieces." [14]
- Emily Ley

Are there areas of your life that stand out as moments where you've fallen? Brokenness that has come from heavier trauma or deeper wounds? You're not alone. Let's move on and consider how we can begin to find hope and wholeness.

Are You Living In Survival Mode?

Maybe for you, the greater challenge is not distraction, but rather it has been a crisis that has affected your confidence. Are you living in survival mode, a constant rush of stress hormones moving through your body as you live each day just to get by, running on the verge of exhaustion? Do you find it challenging to give yourself permission to rest and reflect? Are you fearful of being quiet, still or reflective, unsure of what you might face?

Just a short while ago, while writing this book, we received a late night phone call from our nineteen-year old son. He had been heading home from a business meeting, driving on the interstate between Chicago and Milwaukee when he heard a pop–type explosion and pulled over. He opened the hood to find the engine smoking and on fire! As he ran to the trunk to grab something to try and extinguish the flames, the flames grew larger and the whole situation escalated beyond his control. Backing away, he called 911 and then home, surrendering the situation.

When I arrived and saw the car first-hand, I was astonished at the extent of the damage caused by one little spark under the hood. I was so thankful that he was aware enough to have responded proactively to that initial "pop" because it literally saved his life. How often are we driving our lives when a small spark can pop at any time and engulf our engine in flames? We need to be listening and aware of those little signals that might be telling us that something is getting too hot. Or too empty. Or dangerously eroded. Self-awareness and proper self-care help us discover and prevent destructive habits that can impact our health. This is not only critical to your well-being, but as you will see in later chapters, it is also critical to the well-being of those around you!

"In practicing self-love over the past couple of years, I can say that it has immeasurably deepened my relationships with the people I love."
- Brene Brown

When you're in crisis mode, it takes effort to shift priorities and extend ourselves permission to carve out time for self-care. The silver lining is that self-care can move us out of survival mode into living with intention. Sometimes we get caught in a state of reactive living, aka survival mode, where we are responding by immediate cause and response. You may not feel you have any spare time to carve out for some of these activities. The truth is, taking time for self-care will multiply your efforts and make your time more productive and mindful no matter what that is. Living in survival mode depletes us of our energy stores, our emotional well-being and robs us of depth in our faith. When you fill your bucket with life-giving habits, the less likely you'll fall into feelings of overwhelm and exhaustion. This is a place where you'll likely find better health, more energy and clearer perspectives of your place in the world. The benefits will spill over into all aspects of your life as you live with more focus.

FIGHT/FLIGHT/FREEZE

When you combine daily distractions that are just a part of our modern society with any deeper history of abuse, trauma, being overworked, growing family responsibilities, aging parents, or special needs children, self-care is often forced by the wayside. That is, until that neglect causes a health crisis of its own.

Trauma may thrust us into what can be called a fight/flight/freeze mode, and it can happen to anyone. Trauma doesn't have to be earth shattering to have a profound impact on our bodies; we can carry any type of trauma with us for years in our physical and emotional body. In addition, two people may also respond to similar trauma in very different ways, making the subject of fight/flight/freeze complex.

"Recovery from trauma is to learn to live with the memories of the past without being overwhelmed by them in the present. Just as we need to revisit traumatic memories in order to integrate them, we

need to revisit the parts of ourselves that developed the defensive habits that helped us to survive." [15]
- Bessel Van Der Kolk M.D.

In the simplest explanation, these protective measures were added to our design to protect us during traumatic situations. The problem occurs when we remain in fight/flight/freeze mode beyond the trauma and become disassociated from our emotions and physical body. Secondary trauma can also occur just from witnessing, listening to stories of trauma, reading accounts or seeing them on video. Professionals in mental health, counselors, police officers and loved ones caring for traumatized adults and children can also suffer secondary trauma. I experienced this just weeks after I began researching the atrocities of human trafficking. When I began having nightmares about my research, I realized I needed to step back and shift into more self-care to shield myself from the long term effects of the emotional stress it brought on.

Unmanaged stress and traumatic wounding often lead to similar symptoms:

• Feeling exhausted all the time
• Feeling numb or overwhelmed most days
• Suffering frequent anxiety or panic attacks
• Weakened immune system, getting sick frequently
• Feeling alone and detached

  • Lacking motivation or any sense of accomplishment

Plane Health

If you've ever flown on a plane, you will recall the instructions given just before take-off that in the event of an emergency, you need to secure your own oxygen mask before assisting others. The same is true of self-care. We need to begin with ourselves. If we are stressed out, overwhelmed, or burning the candle at both ends, we are of little help to others. We cannot escape the stresses of life and some things are out of our control, but we can work on our RESPONSES to stress through mindfulness.

The more we identify and take control of our responses when we're under stress, the better our bodies can practice dialing down; this prevents our body from staying in ongoing fight/flight/freeze mode that can result in chronic health issues in the future. You'll learn more about this in later chapters.

"I have needs and I can speak to them - understanding your body helps you unlock and identify what those needs are. Trauma puts us into a place of freeze mode where we shut down and turn off those modes of awareness. Engaging your physical body in sensory experiences can help unlock those fight/flight/freeze modes."
Heidi Vance, Holy Yoga

If I may add a note of encouragement, if you are in an ongoing, broken relationship or harmful situation, you can regain control over your life. Help is available if you choose to reach out for it. If you are determined to walk down a different path in your life and seek deep healing from something you've been experiencing, or feel stuck or helpless, there can be hope and a way out. Look to the resources in the back of this book for more direction and support.

"Step into broken places and start being a part of redemption and resurrection stories."
Ann Voskamp

BUILDING CONFIDENCE

Many people believe that building confidence comes through mastering a talent or having a strong ego through which people can be persuaded. This view of confidence is fed constantly by the millions of hours people spend reading magazines, passing mannequins in the mall, watching TV, videos and movies, all of which idealize success and what it means to be happy and confident. As men, women and children are attracted to and absorb all these images and prototypes, the message the self often receives is that in comparison, it is insufficient, lacking, and of lesser value. The paradox is that comparison through these images is the primary confidence destroyer! Although we can be inspired by other successful people, the illusion of much of what we are seeing has little authentic inspirational value. Imaginary things have imaginary value. Meanwhile, here you are completely real and designed perfectly with a mind, body and spirit! As you begin to be more aware of how you are wired and how you treat each area, you will undoubtedly grow your confidence. The work you do in this space is what will help true healing take place. If one area is messy or devoid of attention, the other areas will lose some of their potential, and your confidence slows. But open up and address that weaker area, applying new wisdom, discernment, and acceptance; and a peace will begin to grow. This is an optimal time to introduce prayer and meditation; as you see and explore the neglect or wound in an area of your life, it can be helpful to rethink what is and isn't important, to forgive yourself, and to seek greater wisdom and support.

I recommend you take a break from media and unplug the noise and constant stimulation. Spend time remembering who you are and what is important to you. It might sound cliche, but in this silence, listen to your body. It will speak, often in aches or shifts in energy, in responses to stimuli you give it through food, rest, emotional and spiritual enlightenment. If you find you feel uncomfortable try and zoom in on what exactly does not feel right, think through your recent history to make connections. Was it the 24-hour flu you just had? Could it be you were exposed to chemicals or unnatural ingredients? Are you agitated from not enough sleep or from a news article you read that stirred up your emotions? Is there a relationship that feels stressful, or a problem that doesn't seem to have an available solution? When you're tuned in to yourself and removed from the constant chatter of technology you might be surprised at how clear the answers might come with practice and observation. This could be called practicing "mindfulness", which is really practicing vigilance. Don Miller writes "You can call it God or a conscience, or you can dismiss it as that intuitive knowing we all have as human beings, but there is a knowing that guides us toward being better."

It will help you discover where you're vulnerable and in need of adjustment so that you can restore your design and your true self. Self-awareness gives us the confidence to make decisions day to day that will build up the fullness of our being and make us less likely to succumb to manipulation by the world, the media, and even our own un-attended thoughts.

Confidence can come from three places: The first is as something we were born with, created to have, (but can also surrender). This core confidence, called authenticity, was wired into our DNA. Secondly, we can also build confidence from outside of ourselves, such as when we master a skill, we build competency in that skill. Mastering the skill isn't what gives us our core confidence in who we were created to be. It definitely adds value to us in feeling like we accomplished something, which is good. When I began writing my blog, I learned how to use my phone for taking pictures and creating inspiring quotes. I gained confidence in using my device to brighten up my social media, but this confidence is limited to my computer use. It really didn't add value to me as a human being, as God's Masterpiece and what He created me to be. I'm glad I learned these skills, but my confidence in who I am runs much deeper than this.

Surrounding ourselves with positive words can keep us focused on doing our best and being our best, but the words are not what create the confidence. These quotes and words can make us feel better and keep our thoughts on the up and up, but they cannot fill in the spaces of poor self-esteem that may have been shaped from a young age or brokenness in our lives (the authenticity that was surrendered). Only we can understand the value of our worth, that is where one source of true confidence lies, which should be independent of our circumstances and experiences. No one can take it away from you and no one else can define it for you if you take responsibility for it and work on it intentionally. The more you depend on your internal confidence the less you'll rely on outside influences to build you up.

"Every time we choose action over ease we develop an increasing level of self-worth, self-respect, and self-confidence." [16]
- John Maxwell, Intentional Living

In being intentional, and not being over-influenced by media, we also know that our confidence can be built by learning new information. The challenge here is finding what information is needed and where is it to be found? We have more information at our fingertips with the ease of the internet than all of recorded history combined! At this rate, it's a very real danger that we are losing sight of the basics in self-care, self-awareness and mindfulness. Our discernment is challenged minute by minute as we filter through thousands of internet sites and online experts every day. Stepping away from all the research, random advice and virtual diagnosing, and instead practicing mindfulness helps you filter through the information overload and make sense of it all.

Self-care involves acting on what you discover through mindfulness, then seeking appropriate fixes based on your value system and where you are in the process. Sometimes things become clear in a moment, but sometimes it takes a while. The beauty is that through regular prayer and meditation, solutions will become clear and your desire to move forward will grow. This is what building confidence is all about. So it becomes merely a matter of time that this new habit of self-examination and meditation coupled with new ideas will help you overcome many obstacles that stand in the way of you reaching your fullest potential.

A major challenge when we learn to listen to ourselves is the problem of the negative and unbelieving voice. There is much written on this subject, but many experts agree that separating out those negative thoughts and excuses, and learning to reframe them for positive application is highly effective. Here are some common negative thoughts many of us experience followed by how we can re-frame them to move us in a better direction:

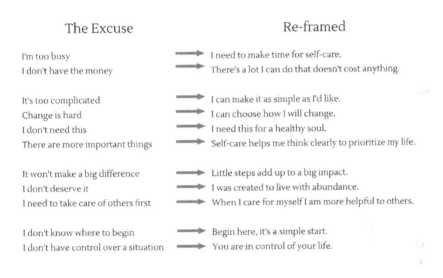

The Excuse	Re-framed
I'm too busy	I need to make time for self-care.
I don't have the money	There's a lot I can do that doesn't cost anything.
It's too complicated	I can make it as simple as I'd like.
Change is hard	I can choose how I will change.
I don't need this	I need this for a healthy soul.
There are more important things	Self-care helps me think clearly to prioritize my life.
It won't make a big difference	Little steps add up to a big impact.
I don't deserve it	I was created to live with abundance.
I need to take care of others first	When I care for myself I am more helpful to others.
I don't know where to begin	Begin here, it's a simple start.
I don't have control over a situation	You are in control of your life.

REFRAMING our thoughts with a positive perspective will give us confidence to move ahead towards healthy choices one small step at a time.

"We have a great deal of worth in the eyes of God. I never tire of saying over and over again that God loves us. It is a wonderful thing that God Himself loves me tenderly. That is why we should have courage, joy and the conviction that nothing can separate us from the love of Christ."[17]
Mother Teresa

Emotional Intelligence and Confidence

Emotional Intelligence is our ability to identify and manage our own emotions as well as being able to understand and respond to other's emotions in a healthy way. Emotional Intelligence is one component in re-framing our perspectives as we "catch" ourselves making excuses day to day. We were created to have a full range of feelings: elation, disappointment, motivation, discouragement, contentment, encouragement, jealousy, anger and hundreds more. All of these emotions were wired into us at birth, but more often than not, they are brought out more by our circumstances and thoughtless reactions than handled properly to benefit ourselves and others. The more we tune into our senses and our feelings, the better we can determine how they influence our life, our past, present or future and look at re-framing our perspectives. If we're feeling vulnerable, anxious or distracted, we may be tempted to look for our confidence in unhealthy places. If we're in control, we stay on track with our mission. When we have mature emotional intelligence versus more primal reactive responsiveness, we can avoid massive fallout in our well-being and relationships.

Emotional Intelligence takes time to develop. It takes practice, stillness, observation and a heart willing to receive truth. Unexpected or traumatic situations can move us into fight/flight/freeze mode which creates an environment in which our emotions swing us like a pendulum within minutes, making it difficult to find middle ground in our responses. Other trauma situations might thrust us into an emotionally numbed state where we have no feelings. When this happens, it's important to take extra time to explore our responses and allow the feelings to surface where they can be addressed. It may help to add these thoughts to your life "story" and record the emotions you've experienced. You may find it helpful to read through Chapter 8: Be Connected through Mind-Body Exercises where there are practical steps you can take to wake up the desensitized and numbed emotions in yourself and learn to feel alive again. Over time, you'll begin to understand how these emotional responses have been shaped over time. If the intensity of the trauma is significant, I would encourage you to seek help in moving from numbness to health once again. Prolonged numbness only leads to self-confusion and disconnection from our mind, body and spirit. When we have clearer understanding of what has influenced us in the past, we can move forward and take loving care of ourselves without giving in to every earthly desire that only satisfies us temporarily.

When we are tuned out of emotional intelligence we may be easily swayed in various situations without realizing it. For example, let's say you call a friend to discuss an important issue and hours or days go by without a return call. This may cause you to feel a range of emotions including anger, neglect, frustration or even abandonment. Any of these feelings may arise because of any number of assumptions: that person doesn't want to talk to me, they are too busy for me, or they intentionally want to offend me. These are all reactive and negative assumptions, when really, it may be that they missed seeing your call. Or they had a crisis that kept them from a normal check in on their phone. If your choice to only think negative thoughts about the silence causes you to become bitter or angry, you risk the relationship and the help. However, with a more mature emotional response, you can find an alternative way to get a hold of that person without getting upset.

Along with emotional intelligence comes greater patience, love and grace with yourself and others because your confidence doesn't rest on outside influences such as whether you receive a return phone call in a set amount of time. When we give ourselves grace in the range of emotions we might have and create space to observe those emotions and decide how we will respond in any given situation we allow our confidence to remain in truth rather than be led by circumstances. This is the place we can extend grace to those around us and take time to see good intentions and motives in others as we have ourselves. The more we understand why we do what we do, the more we see why others behave the way they do without assigning hurtful motives. People everywhere are crying out for the world to be more compassionate and understanding. Emotional intelligence gives us the insight to extend that compassion to those around us.

Building confidence and cultivating self-awareness in the small things such as our emotions day to day will help us become more authentic and healthy over time. When we take charge of constructing our own confidence, it builds roots that anchor deeper - and to the soul, this matters! Building confidence is always active and because of that, it will saturate our decision-making, helping align our priorities and eventually leading us to change our perspectives so that every part of our life aligns with what we care about.

At this point, our confidence gains what is called "moral authority". Moral authority can be based on principles, or fundamental truths, which are independent of our written laws. Moral authority requires us to adhere to those principles regardless of our emotions. When our motives, our moral compass, and the truest form of ourselves are aligned in our mind, our physical body, and our spirit, we can have confidence to move ahead in peace, purpose and continuity. This is not achieving a point of perfection, of striving to get ahead, but rather a continuous peace knowing we are headed in the right direction toward truth. Aligning all elements of ourselves brings in grace, self-acceptance and love that we can also extend to those around us in all that we do. We can continue to grow in grace when we extend that authentic love from ourselves to those around us.

Having said all of this on the subject of confidence, we can see that developing better self-esteem is a process and it takes vigilance. However, because we are imperfect, sometimes broken people, and the goal line for perfection is beyond any horizon, we still have a problem. There is one final confidence available to us, and it comes completely externally, one in which we must become completely dependent on something greater than ourselves as I have found in the One True God. This confidence comes through grace, knowing that He loves us and has our best interest in mind.

When we choose to receive this grace, it multiplies everything in our life for good because the grace comes from outside of us.

We can put aside all of our earthly expectations or experiences of what God may or may not be, because above all things, He knows us better that we even know ourselves. He is the one who designed us and has plans for us. Under this banner we live our lives. Under this banner, ask yourself:

· Why do I do what I do?

· Why do I believe what I believe?

If you want to really embrace your life and move ahead in confidence, asking these questions is a necessary component. You may not be able to answer these right away. Understanding exactly what you believe often comes slowly as you peel away layers that have formed through human interactions and experiences, good and bad. Discovering grace from God and gaining His perspective can be the missing link that can pull everything together, but it's a gift you need to receive.

The One True God is a god of invitation. In the book of Matthew, Jesus invites us to look for answers, to discover what we might not even realize we need: "Ask and it will be given to you, seek and you will find; knock and the door will be opened to you. For everyone who asks receives; he who seeks finds; and to him who knocks, the door will be opened."[18] He offers us a sanctuary of grace as He invites us: "Come to me all who are weary and burdened, and I will give you rest."[19] In Psalm 91:1 He brings us into the fullness of His grace and invites us to enter into a place of security, to live in the realm of God: "he who dwells in the shelter of the Most High will rest in the shadow of the Almighty." [20] Whatever you place your beliefs in will shape how your confidence grows.

Chapter 4: Building Purpose

Living With Discipline and Intention

Discipline is the beginning point of any positive change as we determine what should be done to improve and moving ahead regardless of how we "feel" about it. As you discover various courses of action (wellness tools) here and as you move forward in life, write them down somewhere so that you can be reminded of what works with your personality, values and personal vision. That is the beginning of being intentional, which leads to discipline.

 All intention and discipline must begin with a personal vision and subsequent goals if the work is to be meaningful. Without an endpoint or compass to guide us, it can be easy to put components of our life into individual categories and miss the goals we hope to achieve. Ephesians 5:16 instructs us to "Make the most of every opportunity"; however, what if every waking moment provides us with countless opportunities? We can easily fill up our days with "good opportunities" that lead us down unproductive paths that distract us from the few great things that really count. An opportunity to work-out Sunday through Saturday, to join the book club on Tuesdays, to volunteer at the pet shelter Thursday night, to attend church on Sunday, Wednesday and Saturday mornings, Facebook events, school activities, support groups not only busy us, they also makes it easy to compartmentalize our lives into separate ventures that distract the goal.

Operating our lives in compartmentalized fashion without a personal mission statement puts us at risk of overextending ourselves. When we operate with consideration of our own personal path, we can experience not less, but greater satisfaction and growth. An abundance mentality begins to emerge where once a scarcity of time/energy once existed. It truly bears repeating that without a clear purpose, we have no foundation on which we base decisions, allocate time, and use resources. We will tend to make choices based on circumstances, pressures, and the mood of the moment. People who don't know their purpose try to do too much, and that causes stress, fatigue, and conflict.[21]

"We should never underestimate the significance of what we think about ourselves, the calling and purpose we hold on to that drives our lives forward. What is it that gets you out of bed in the morning? What is your personal vision for your life?"[22]

In the Bible, we are told that God has a plan and a purpose for our lives if we *seek it* and follow after Him. This is when His perfect intentions can become our intentions to live with abundance. When we let go of following random earthly desires we create contentment in our life.

The Purpose of a Purpose

Motivation will be the driving force behind making positive changes in your life. Inspiration and encouragement can come from others and how they are living their life, but only you can determine how much thought and energy you are willing to put into changing your life. In order to find honest motivation, your biggest challenge will be finding the most important reason(s) behind your desire to change. This is what is meant by finding your "WHY". These motivators tend to fall in 3 categories:

- Material or physical
- Recognition and accomplishment
- Legacy or Cause-driven

Do you want to feel better physically? Would you like healthier relationships with others? Would having more success at your job be meaningful? Do you seek a deeper faith that changes not only you, but influences others? Once you know your "WHY", you'll have direction and fuel to motivate you. If your why isn't defined, you'll most likely fall into the energy of other people's "WHY", surrendering your authenticity, purpose, and ultimately, your joy.

"Your call provides you with your life direction. It informs your decisions by reorienting your priorities and establishing a new set of core values. Your call provides a content that becomes your life message. You will not be who you are without it."
- Reggie McNeal

How to Begin Discovering Your "Why"

One way to begin the discovering how you are motivated is start by listing the things you most love to do, things from which you derive enjoyment and peace. Sometimes these activities correspond with your gifts, so you will want to consider that. Often as we get older and take on more responsibilities, we forget things we used to enjoy; think back on your life to times when you spent hours doing things you loved, or recall a memory that always brings you joy. Recalling things for this list may take some time, so keep a notebook or journal nearby and capture those thoughts for a few days/weeks. Set a goal to find 10 things you truly have enjoyed and record them here:

Next you'll want to survey where you are **at this time** in your life. It will be difficult to create a plan to move forward if you aren't aware of where you are. There are likely some areas of your life that you are more satisfied and confident about than others, and that is okay. Being balanced in every area is a goal, but acknowledging where you are now is healthy in that you can begin to find inspiration to change the areas with which you are less satisfied. The goal is not perfection, nor is perfection the bar. The greatest satisfaction you will find is in the journey of personal growth. It may sound cliché, but when you are seeing changes in yourself, it becomes its own reward.

On a scale of 1 -,10 rate yourself in the following areas. (1 being weak to non-existant and 10 being a model example):

_____   1. Spiritual – a relationship with God inclusive of worship, prayer and spiritual Engagement

_____   2. Family – bonds and relationships with both immediate and extended members

_____   3. Work – performing your vocation, career, job or volunteer work

_____   4. Education – an on-going practice of learning new things or digging deeper

_____   5. Creativity – outlets for hobbies, arts, leisure practices

_____   6. Physical – attention to health, physical movement/exercise, strength and flexibility

_____   7. Organizational – prioritizing and scheduling events, people and rest/leisure

_____   8. Leisure – developing and practicing hobbies

_____   9. Financial - developing a short-term and long-term plan for money

Now ask yourself the following questions combining your thoughts on what you most enjoy and your level of satisfaction in these 9 areas (journaling your answers):

1.   Would I like to learn more about having a stronger faith? What has held me back from pursuing this? What would I like my faith/spiritual life to look like?

2.   Would I like to be a catalyst for change in my family? What attitudes do I currently have that prevent me from serving and enjoying my family? What would I like my family life to look like?

3.   Is what I am doing to earn money now something I consider a

job, a career, or a calling? Do I want to continue doing what I am doing, or do I feel called to do something else? If I could do anything with my days, what would I like to do?

4.   Would I like to become a strong learner at this point in my life? Why did I(if I have) stop learning? What are things I would love to learn about?

5.   Would I like more time or resources for a creative outlet? What area of creativity attracts me the most? If I could really excel in a creative endeavor, what would that area be?

6.   Would I like to become a healthier person? What holds me back from practicing good health habits such as exercise, diet, relaxation or proper physical healing?

7.   Would I like to be a more organized person? What habits do I have that create distraction/confusion or chaos in my life? What would a well-planned day look like for me?

8.   Would I like more time for leisure for myself or with other people? What prevents me from scheduling leisure activities? What activities would I love to do more consistently?

9.   Would I like to have better financial fitness? What is my greatest financial challenge? If finances were handled and I were financially free, what would I do with my life?

Your Personal Mission Statement

The next step in discovering your "why" is to create a personal mission statement To do this, you will need to clarify the things you most value with how you like to do things and what your gifts are. Lastly you will tie in what you desire to see done. This three-step process of discovering your mission is simple but effective. Take time to think deeply about this. When you are done, you should be able to see clearly what your mission in life may be.

First, to clarify the things you value the most, consider the following list. Ask yourself for each one, "how important is this?" 1 being the least important, 5 being something you couldn't operate without. I would say......[23]

Honesty	1	2	3	4	5
Freedom	1	2	3	4	5
Justice	1	2	3	4	5
Courage	1	2	3	4	5
Hunger	1	2	3	4	5
Success	1	2	3	4	5
Fairness	1	2	3	4	5
Flexibility	1	2	3	4	5
Recognition	1	2	3	4	5
Peace	1	2	3	4	5
Worship	1	2	3	4	5
Faith	1	2	3	4	5
Integrity	1	2	3	4	5
Tradition	1	2	3	4	5
Power	1	2	3	4	5
Friendship	1	2	3	4	5
Security	1	2	3	4	5
Wealth	1	2	3	4	5
Legacy	1	2	3	4	5
Joy	1	2	3	4	5
Family	1	2	3	4	5
Health	1	2	3	4	5
Acceptance	1	2	3	4	5
Career	1	2	3	4	5
Excellence	1	2	3	4	5
Fame	1	2	3	4	5
Influence	1	2	3	4	5
Truth	1	2	3	4	5

Goetschel, Chuck. Simon Says. Obstacles Press, Inc. Grand Blane, Michigan. 2009.

Next, go back and list all those that have the highest score (5).

Of those you listed as scoring the highest, choose the top 6 that you could never be without.

Of your top 6, choose which 3 you would preserve for all the generations after you. Rank them #1, #2, and #3.

FINISH THE FOLLOWING SENTENCES:

The three things I value the most are #1_____ #2 _____ and #3_____.

#1_____: to me, having success in this area means_____.

#2_____: to me, having success in this area means_____.

#3_____: to me, having success in this area means_____.

What you have done is just defined success in your top three chosen core values! Now you need only to put all three values together in a single short paragraph beginning with "Success in my life means….." and follow it with your three answers.

Your calling is linked to your desires and your gifts. Let's take a moment to explore some potential gifts. Circle 3 to which you are most attracted:

organizing	inspiring	traveling
comforting	leading	exploring
mentoring	encouraging	negotiating
inventing	solving	persuading
managing	writing	caring
analyzing	uplifting	reading
clarifying	healing	entertaining
researching	teaching	coaching
speaking	repairing	other
building	supporting	

Desire: Which of these activities do I desire and feel I am naturally gifted at doing?

Value: When people come to me, what are they wanting to receive from me? What do I provide for them?

Success: When I recall a successful experience in my life, what was it I contributed?

Putting It All Together

Using your answers from above, finish the following statement:

My calling is to be (your desire and gifts):

Success in my life as I do this will look like (#1, #2 and #3 above).

Now that you have specifics written down, you can be more disciplined in decisions you face and intentional in the choices you make. Every decision you make with your time, energy and resources will either take you closer to your calling and goals or farther from them. Find someone who can help you remain accountable in moving in that direction.

Who can support me in reaching my personal goals? Who are the influencers in my life?

Hopefully what you are learning in discovering your purpose is that you can begin to think bigger about yourself and your life's purpose. If we want to create healthy perspectives such as the glass is half full versus half empty, we should look at opportunities for growth rather than focusing on the obstacles to getting us there. When we integrate all areas of our life to align with our purpose we can bring together the mind, body and spirit.

How often do we limit our own abundance by living out our lives in compartments, scarcity and fear? We put our faith in one box, health in another and emotional stability in yet another and long to live a life of purpose. In the process we might end up feeling fragmented, isolated or unsatisfied in the spaces of our lives where there should be abundance. Combining all areas into the same box not only maximizes the positive impact in each area, it brings simplicity to our lives and a cohesiveness that helps put all our choices in perspective. **We are not just randomly making decisions for health, wellness, relationships and faith, but integrating them all together to work towards the same goals, fulfilling our purpose here on Earth** so we can be in fellowship with others and share God's love with those around us. This is how we can discover God-sized abundance.

"For I know the plans I have for you", declares the Lord, "plans to prosper you and not harm you, plans to give you hope and a future."
Jeremiah 29:11

Because you will find your spirit and faith are most fed when you are living intentionally, I would encourage you to take these exercises and thoughts to prayer. Pray daily that God would help you use your time, your energy, your gifts, your resources, your desires and even your struggles to help you fulfill your purposes. Reading biographies, stories or scripture about others who lived intentionally will also inspire you to do the same. There are countless worthy examples of people living and in the pages of history whom you can look to for courage and faithfulness. Ask the people in your life whom you respect the most who they find inspiring if you are unsure where to begin. I guarantee you will truly enjoy this discovery!

Chapter 5: Building a Healthy Spirit and Body Image

THE STARTING AND ENDING POINT OF REALLY LIVING

Discovering Solitude: Be Still and Know I am God

Are you comfortable with quiet? Do you feel restless or uneasy when you're still? If so, you are not alone. I was for many years! If you came into my home, you would have found the television or radio on constantly. Sometimes I would have the volume so loud that I couldn't hear my own thoughts above it. I grew up with a busy childhood with a lot of opportunities and activities and not a lot of time for reflection. As a result, I didn't really understand myself well. I was caught up in busyness but lacked time to process the things I was experiencing. In my teen years, the busyness led to destructive habits that further numbed my introspection. I also experienced some trauma that led to years of depression and an eating disorder. The last thing I wanted to experience was any kind of stillness that would force me to face all of that! I might have replayed unpleasant events or come face to face with my own selfish thoughts and poor decisions. No thank you!

Psalm 46:10 begins, "Be still and know that I am God". It was when I began to seek and know God that I gradually became more comfortable with the "still" part. By opening my heart and mind to begin discovering who God is, I was changed. Grace washed over me as I found a new faith and extended forgiveness to myself. I repented of my destructive habits; that is, I acknowledge them and turned away from them. God, through his Holy Spirit created a new space in my life, one in which I could now rest in solitude. I was introduced to Yoga which gave me practical tools to connect my physical body and mind with stillness. These practices have made all the difference for me and it's the reason I'm a wellness advocate today. Because of this transformation, my passion is not just teaching healthy eating and exercise, but integrating these routines gently into the mind and soul as well.

"Our body houses not only the Holy Spirit Himself, but the heart, will, mind, and emotions-all that plays a part in our knowing God and living for Him."
-Elisabeth Elliot

Stillness provides us the space to think about what we're doing, and discover why we do what we do. You can find hope in the stillness even if all seems hopeless, scary or overwhelming. The grace of the Holy Spirit releases you of fear. 2 Timothy 1:7 says, "for God gave us a spirit not of fear but of power and love and self-control". Running from stillness will not make our troubles go away. Real change can only begin when you face the truths in your life, accept them and move ahead in another direction. What you will find is every experience and choice you've had adds to your wisdom. Understanding ourselves better through stillness helps us to see where we are influenced by circumstances, media and the people around us. It allows us to hear the most important voice.

"God made our souls to long for Him, and we are not fully satisfied without His presence in our lives."
- Beth Moore

When we allow God's Holy Spirit to reveal these things to us, we will be lovingly convicted to follow Him and the purpose He has for our life. Living with this kind of daily reflection results in a very sweet spot of self-care in which you receive what you truly need, emotionally, physically, and spiritually. You will find a sense of belonging, abundance and value the world cannot give.

Would you like to receive direction from God in your life? Receive the grace, love, wisdom and strength to live out your life with Him? The invitation is always available to anyone who wants to receive it.

"Therefore, I urge you, brothers and sisters, in view of God's mercy, to offer your bodies as a living sacrifice, holy and pleasing to God - this is your true and proper worship. Do not conform to the pattern of this world, but be transformed by the renewing of your mind. Then you will be able to test and approve what God's will is - his good, pleasing and perfect will."

Romans 12:1-2

Practicing Worship

We all worship something. Worship is defined as 1. reverence paid to merit or worth; respect; adoration to God or a sacred object. 2. to adore. Anything can become an object of worship if it is elevated above everything else in our hearts, it's whatever we value.[24] Therefore, make your worship matter for what counts the most. If God has you in the palm of his hand and loves you beyond human understanding, He is showing you his heart. For these reasons and more, He is worthy of your worship. Your response to this truth is an act of worship. Spending time contemplating this, reading Scripture, thanking Him for his goodness, and enjoying Him is pure worship. This is what God enjoys as well! The togetherness you find with Him in these moments truly purifies your life and blesses not only you, but all those around you.

The choices we make in our lives define who or what we worship.

When you choose to receive the gift of Jesus, you'll discover a clearer calling and direction in your life that will define your "why". This direction will guide your decisions by reorienting their priorities and establishing a new set of core values. The call provides a content that becomes your life message. You will not be who you are without it.[25]

Finding safety through stillness and rest

It's amazing all of the ways we try to fill our instinctual hunger for personal wholeness by searching outside ourselves. Because we don't feel whole or satisfied, we conclude that we are not competent or intuitive enough to feel "put together" and so the search begins. It is as if this desire is supernaturally broadcasted into the airwaves and thousands of companies and opportunists spring into action to make known to us the miracle product or service we can purchase to solve all of our problems. Yet the paradox is that often, we don't even know the real problem that all these products and people are trying to solve.

"Some of your great heart hungers may still be unsatisfied. God may be using these to create space for himself in your heart. As long as you look to others, to achievement, or to anything but God to fill the void, the hunger will be your master."
Reggie McNeal

The reason we have a longing is because we have questions that are not yet answered. No product is effective unless it solves a specific problem. Bad habits are formed when we don't take time to address the real problem and instead, use, or should I say mis-use things to ignore, mute, stuff, deny or refuse them. When we do this, we end up in a less safe, more confused state. Instead, we need to go back to the source of the One who made us, our Creator, and see what He has to say about it. The Bible is very clear on the hungers of the human soul and what can make us whole again. When we ask him,

Jesus himself promises he will answer. In fact in the Bible, there is a recounting of a time Jesus made himself available to a woman who had this very hunger to feel complete:

As Jesus was traveling though Samaria on is way to Galilee, he stopped at a well while his disciples went to town for food. A Samaritan woman came to the same well to draw water, and Jesus asked her for a drink. This woman was quite surprised that Jesus was even talking to her because Jews typically did not talk or associate with Samaritans.

Jesus replied, "If you knew the gift of God and who it is that asks you for a drink, you would have asked him and he would have given you living water." This caused the woman to ask where someone would get living water like that! So Jesus went on to say "Everyone who drinks this water will be thirsty again, but whoever drinks the water I give them will never thirst. Indeed, the water I give them will become in them a spring of water welling up to eternal life."

That sounded amazing to the woman who pictured not having to go to a well every day to draw water. She seemed very weary.

Next, Jesus asked her to get her husband, to which she replied she had no husband. Jesus, being fully God as well as fully man knew this about her, and he knew she actually had five husbands and was now just living with a man. This knowledge surprised the woman further and she began sensing Jesus was no ordinary man for in addition to promising her living water, he also pointed to her deepest pain. Jesus had completely drawn her in, and in that freedom she began to ask about hope…hope in a Messiah who would someday come and explain why she and the world around her were so broken. then Jesus declared, "I, the one speaking to you- I am he." John 4:3-26

Did you catch what she was hungering and thirsting for? She wanted a husband that met her needs, she wanted certainty, truth, something to believe in. And Jesus merely pointed out that anything you take externally from the world will leave you thirsting. This is also what I want you to consider. Before you embark on the many fixes we have for broken parts of our lives, first consider seeking spiritual wholeness from a God who will supply it from within you. And when the soul is satisfied, your perspective on all other areas of your life will change, altering the quality of the decisions you make. Your standard and decision making will be truth and not convenience, leading to lasting change and healing. Without truth and the influence of God's lordship in your life, you will be as a vineyard invaded by foxes, or as the Bible says, open to thieves who come to steal and destroy.

So what is it we hunger for that will be revealed in stillness? Ravi Zacharias details it best:

"If we were to enumerate all our hungers, we might be surprised at how many legitimate hungers there are. The hunger for truth, the hunger for love, the hunger for knowledge, the hunger to belong, the hunger to express, the hunger for justice, the hunger of the imagination, the hunger of the mind, and the hunger for significance. We could name more. Not only do we remain unfulfilled when we pursue these hungers, but in their very pursuit comes a disorientation that misrepresents and misunderstands where the real satisfaction comes from."[26]

Practicing self-awareness by being still gives us the opportunity to develop skills that can identify valid hungers versus hungers that lead to destructive pitfalls. We'll find that some of our hungers are not bad in and of themselves, and some are actually clues to feeling more whole. Others are clues to wants that the world may have convinced us of as false needs. If we don't take time to sort these hungers or if we confuse them, the world hungers can gain strength, often manifesting themselves in states of fatigue, grief, dissatisfaction, despair, depression and loneliness. These are dangerous imbalances because they can result in weaknesses in our character as we are more vulnerable to making poor choices. Anything that creates confusion in our lives makes it more challenging to see beyond our immediate circumstances; confusion works against orderly and principled decision-making, increasing the likelihood that our stability and safety will be compromised in some way.

Rest

Similar to stillness is rest. Where stillness is defined as absence of motion to seek new thoughts, rest is breaking from stress or busyness to a slower pace or full stop to discontinue everything and just be. A good rest gives us the opportunity to heal and detoxify our physical body; the brain decreases it's activity and diverts blood flow to repair cells damaged by muscle use, breakdown and production of stress hormones. The body literally resets itself with good rest so that when done, it can return to optimal functioning. When rest is sleep, hormones are released which stimulates tissue growth and muscle repair, our immune system primes itself to defend against infection and foreign invaders. When rest is relaxation, we emotionally reset and gain distance between ourselves and the stresses we experience. Relaxation provides us opportunities to understand our perspectives. Situations seem different after a good night's sleep, a weekend away, or a change of pace. The crowded responses we experience under stress are parted and we can come at the issues with new strength and inspiration to reframe, solve or manage problems. And sometimes it is even better to rest just before we enter into stillness!

Everyone experiences occasional days of unrest, lost sleep or difficulty building in stillness to our days. Chronic loss of these important components of self-care though can wreak havoc on our physical body, affect our concentration and healthy brain function and distract us from our spiritual selves and our feelings of safety and security. I went through a season of fatigue which attacked my feelings of wholeness in all of these ways. After my first son was born, like many newborns, he had an ever-changing sleep pattern. I found myself waking earlier and earlier to his cries, sometimes waking at on or two-o'clock in the morning. I endured months of sleep deprivation before we finally found a solution to his erratic sleeping patterns. This lack of sleep gave me a mind filled with confusion - a real fog. I found myself being more impulsive and irritable, something that affected the dynamics of our whole family. This also caused great stress in my physical body and my spirit. It was not much different than previous emotional trauma I had experienced in my life. Weariness in any of the areas of mind, body and spirit may look much the same, whether it's illness, drug abuse, trauma, or emotional strongholds. You can be robbed of feelings of safety and security. When you are caught in the confusion of your situation, it can be difficult to understand the hungers that are genuine versus those that are brought on by skewed circumstances.

Rest can also come after release, specifically release from anger and guilt. Whether we have been wronged or we are responsible for a wrong, the stress and turmoil this causes prevents the kind of peace we seek. Learning to forgive others is a powerful skill, and to learn more about that, I would encourage you to find a mentor or a counselor to walk you through it. But forgiving yourself is something I want to address here. In our rest and in our stillness, as we find ourselves periodically recalling poor choices we've made, we can take the same opportunity to view that choice as something of the past and close it off by forgiving ourselves. This process is called repentance, which is admitting what we have done and at the same time admitting it was not something we wanted to do and will then turn away from doing it again. It allows us to consider offering apologies to ourselves or to others whom we may have hurt. It is soul work, releasing guilt, shame or disappointment from our in-most self.

"Notice that rest comes AFTER repentance. We must repent and then we

MUST REST. Refreshment comes in the Lord. We repent…we give. Then we rest…we receive. Rest is immensely important so that we give God time to lay a new foundation in our hearts and in our minds. A new truth in the soil of that which repentance made space for. We exchange the lies we live for the TRUTH about who God IS and who we are in relationship to His being Lord of our lives."
-Brook Boone, Holy Yoga

Repentance comes when we fully lay down those strongholds of poor decisions or habits so that positive change can be cultivated in our spirit. In the Christian faith, repentance is most important to God who extends the fullness of His grace when we forgive ourselves as He forgives us. In the book of Biblical book of the Psalms, David writes "I will lie down and sleep in peace, for you alone, O God, make me dwell in safety." Safety in this verse translates as a refuge, security and feeling of trust. Would you like to experience more safety in your life? would you consider that God cares about you and wants to support you as you heal and care for yourself in many ways? When you receive forgiveness from Him, you also receive the ultimate gifts of grace, security, peace and acceptance.

Pick up a FREE copy of the Mindfulness Mapping ebook: 25 questions to ask yourself for better understanding of your Perceptions, Priorities and Personality.

http://bit.ly/MINDFULNESSmapping

Breathing In Stillness and Rest

In the journey to discover more about ourselves physically, emotionally and spiritually through stillness and rest, we have a tool so powerful it can literally change everything in moments. Learning the art of breathing can change your physical responses, your mental clarity, and your emotional energy. It has strong applications in body movement as you'll see in the chapter on stretching and yoga exercises. It is a simple but essential body function that can either inhibit our body's performance or enhance it, and it's something you can use for increased wellness no matter where you are. Breath gives life. Breath is the space where we can find more understanding. Breath is the space where we can pause and see just how we are in that moment - physically, emotionally, spiritually.

Then he took a deep breath and breathed into them. "Receive the Holy Spirit," he said. [27]

Harnessing the power of breathing is fairly easy to do, it just takes practice and intention. It begins with awareness much like everything else we've discussed. Begin by tuning-in to how easily you're breathing at any moment. Are you slow and relaxed? Are you taking deeper breaths than normal or sighing? Are you finding you're holding your breath in a protective way? In each breath we are bringing oxygen into the lungs, where hemoglobin helps it move into the bloodstream. From there it moves on to the heart which pumps it to the rest of the body. By speeding up or slowing down this process, you speed up or slow down oxygenation to your organs, muscles, nerves, and protective tissues. When you learn to control your breath patterns, you control the relationship between your body and mind by creating more energy (oxygenation), lessening energy, or interrupting energy. You can see how this can be very powerful and empowering!

I recently had some dental work done that required anesthesia and some drilling. You see, I'm paying later in life for my younger years when I enjoyed eating far too many Charleston Chews candies. My old fillings have been breaking down and were in need of replacing, a routine I've undergone before. Because I was familiar with the procedure I could anticipate my anesthesia wearing off a little soon before the job was finished. I found myself frozen a number of times, stuck on an inhale. Each time I caught myself holding my breath, I relaxed my shoulders and took a few deep breathes to get back on track. I knew what to do, but my body had been caught in a breath-holding pattern from past experiences. My awareness helped me to move out of those holding patterns more quickly so my body and mind could move into intentional relaxation techniques until the procedure was done. Keeping my body and mind relaxed was an important step in supporting my body in healing from the trauma of the dental work. My awareness helped me break old thought patterns and observe how the emotional anxiousness of the situation was causing me to hold my breath.

Learning breath control can also enhance athletic or artistic performances. For example, many musicians have used their breath as a tool to improve their concentration, mental clarity, and understanding of their work. Simply timing our breath pattern with a piece of calming music is an easy way to regulate our breathing. Inhaling an equal amount of time that we exhale. Zita Zohar is an internationally renowned concert pianist and master teacher. She instructs that regulating breath with the music helps to "organize the brain and body to move in tandem with the music."[28] When our breath patterns are more regular, it helps all our body systems work more efficiently, especially our brain. Our breath regulation creates healthier brain functioning that can give us clear perspectives and influence how we perceive our selves in the world.

In summary, taking time to cultivate clearer perspectives, personal feelings of safety and a strong sense of purpose depends on the awareness we have of our needs for stillness and rest. When we carve out time in our schedule for quiet and restoration we can be more focused and deliberate in everything we do, including what we think about ourselves.

The most basic self-awareness we can have is of our breath. Because we rely on it all day long we have endless opportunities to engage it and improve insight into our body in a simple, practical way.

Creating a Positive Body Image

The last 'Core Connection" that is essential to laying a foundation for a healthier you is the mindset of a healthy body image. Loving and accepting ourselves is at the core of a positive body image, but how do we make that happen? How do we sort through what we actively tell ourselves and what we've passively been messaged? We all have had our lifetime of influences in this area, and to a lesser or greater degree, it's shaped our self-worth. What hangs in the balance is what we consider beautiful, what creates confidence and how we perceive our place in this world. That's why we need to address this as a core belief.

Everyone is tattered and torn in some way, most often we wear the brokenness and carry it with us everywhere we go, unaware, even forgetting the roots of where it might have began. Or maybe it's always right in front of you, the brokenness that you feel you'll never escape. You can find beauty in the brokenness. Redemption. Because you always have DIGNITY. It's never left you, it just needs to be revealed again, repaired and restored to it's divine structure. We have a choice as to how we will reveal that dignity if it may be hidden.

One of the most empowering and inspiring attitudes we can have about ourselves is found in the word DIGNITY. When we see this trait in others, we almost feel as if there is a deep value and cause about them. How is your personal dignity? How is your truth filter as worldly messages come at you through the internet, media and society? Does your self-dignity rub off on the world around you, or does the world around you attack your dignity? You are an amazing masterpiece, designed for good things in this world; nothing can change the potential you have to be a light in this world! You intrinsically have great dignity, the truth of that is found in some scripture of the Bible:

"For you created my inmost being; you knit me together in my mother's womb. I praise you because I am fearfully and wonderfully made. Your works are wonderful, I know that full well. My frame was not hidden from you when I was made in the secret place. When I was woven together in the depths of the earth, your eyes saw my unformed body."
Psalm 139:13-16

We have a choice to embrace dignity and not fall into a victim mindset no matter what our circumstances are. Dignity calls us to move ahead in confidence to do what we believe is right for ourselves and those around us regardless of how other's might try to tear us down. Dignity claims that deep confidence in the recesses of our heart and mind that no one and no situation can steal. Every human being deserves dignity.

Every person deserves respect. It's no mystery that our culture worships the glamorous and the beautiful without revealing the damage it does to our self-images. Encouragingly, the many voices pouring in over social media and blogs seem be countering the Hollywood message of "sex sells" as people are tired of unattainable standards. However, there are still plenty of messages that fill outdoor advertising spaces and graphic images in clothing stores for us to content. Surrounding ourselves with positivity is a great way to focus on our real worth and build healthy self-esteem. Surrounding ourselves with other's who bring out the best in us will also help support that healthy body image. But we also need to take a look inside for messages there, too. What are you presented with when you look at yourself in the mirror? How deep or how shallow are the thoughts your own image presents to you?

"Mirror, mirror on the wall who's the fairest of them all?" Snow White aired in movie theaters in 1937 so we can hardly deny the prevalence and emphasis of beauty in the public sector for many decades. Mirrors really do nothing but objectively give us our reflection, but how often do we take that image and bundle it with dissatisfaction, guilt, or even hatred? Hopefully, there are times when you smile at what you see! Or maybe one day, you are content with how you are feeling, only to see yourself in the mirror the next day and be reminded of a physical flaw. Any woman knows the insecurity that surfaces in the fitting room of a favorite store when you're trying on swimsuits - too many mirrors and some unflattering lighting create a stressful situation for self-esteem no matter how fit you are! (What potential there is for retailers to improve that experience!)

Mirror, mirror....

After my husband's accident, he endured countless surgeries to repair 3rd degree burns that covered over 50% of his body. Not only are severe burns painful beyond words, they leave scars. Before my husband returned home from the hospital I wanted to eliminate any extra mirrors in our house to protect him from the secondary trauma of seeing disfigurement. Eventually, yes, he was going to have to face his scars and accept them as part of who he was. Over time, he learned to see himself again beyond the scars and is able to focus on others, ministering to, serving, and leading people of all ages. It would have been a tragedy if my husband's self-image came only from what he saw in the mirror versus what he saw in God's mirror. Keeping all our focus on the scars (physical or emotional) of our past only holds us back from the purpose of why we are here - the purpose that makes us all beautiful.

Body image almost always begins with how we feel about our size and weight. There was a season in my life I ditched my scale because of these two culprits. The fact is, our size and weight may vary greatly over our lifetime, but that doesn't need to affect our self-image. I've learned now to perceive my weight based on how my clothes fit and how healthy I feel. If you find you get pre-occupied with mirrors or the numbers on the scale, may I suggest you consider removing them even for a period of time? Building a healthy body image can begin when you focus more on your heart condition, thoughts and emotions. Give yourself a boost in confidence and tuck the mirrors away.

"In solitude you discover a sense of your own beauty. No one else can see the world as you do or sense yourself as you do or feel your life as you do. This is where real beauty lies. There is an intimate connection between the way we look at things and what we actually discover. If you can learn to look at yourself and your life in a gentle, creative, and adventurous way, you will be eternally surprised at what you find."[29]

Body image by nature is also a privacy issue, bringing us to two more considerations: modesty and sexuality. Modesty is the boundary of what you would consider viewable for public and what would be concealed for private. Marketing campaigns glamorize the exposure of skin as shorts creep shorter and clothes fit tighter. The ongoing conversation about where it's acceptable to wear yoga pants is not about limiting personal freedom or putting a heavy burden on individuals about expectations of appropriate clothing, but rather about what is our modern definition of modesty. The core message in all of it is where are we looking for acceptance? What are we willing to do to follow trends? If we lose sight of what is acceptable dress for certain situations, who decides what is appropriate? For job interviews? Awards ceremonies? How can we display respect for a situation or towards an individual by the way we dress? As a culture, how will this lack of direction affect us all as individuals in other areas of our life? Where do you draw the line, if any? Do you value modesty in clothing? Do you think about it? Be gentle with yourself and use some of your quiet time to reflect and understand how trends influence you and how you feel about your body, specifically how you clothe and protect it.

Nothing reveals how we feel about our bodies more than our individual sexuality. Dignity plays a huge role here again as does beauty and purpose. I love the term "Beauty Secrets" that was once referred to in skin care commercials, but is really an essence of our human sexuality. The word "beauty" reminds us that there is goodness and purpose for this aspect of our selves. The word "secrets" means it is deeply personal and requires trust to share. 'Beauty Secrets' are the most sacred parts of our body. In the Bible, God instructs us to save these secrets for a marriage relationship between a man and a woman. He identifies the marriage relationship as so sacred that it is included in the Ten Commandments, the foundational directions for an abundant life. God's intention is that we experience an order and directions for our sexuality, one that brings joy and pleasure, peace and security. Much of the pain, abuse, and brokenness people experience sexually is because this order God intended is violated or compromised. He wants us to see ourselves as temples of the Holy Spirit, as valuable gifts intended to live peaceably and to honor Him, ourselves, and our spouses.

There are many excellent, faith-filled books published on the subject of healthy sexuality, but I'd like to mention just a few core thoughts:

1. Respecting and caring for your body's health through daily care and regular check-ups allows you to prevent problems and to have frequent opportunities to notice any potential problems. This is not only healthy, it is something you deserve.
2. Respect and protect your eyes and mind from unhealthy images and scenes. "The eye is the lamp of the body. If your eyes are healthy, your whole body will be full of light. But if your eyes are unhealthy, your whole body will be full of darkness." Matthew 6:22-23.
3. Handle social media with care. We lose the sacred when our respect for the sacred has vanished. Modern technology destroys the private if we let it.

4. Constantly remind yourself that your body is a temple of the Holy Spirit and requires goodness and order.

Of course, there are many situations that have resulted in divorce, abuse, and trauma that have violated our sacred spaces. Your 'beauty secrets' are a gift, but our modern culture has diminished the pricelessness of this treasure. Women and men who have given away these treasure so easily often fall into a lifetime of searching for self-esteem in places that may never deliver true confidence. If your treasures were taken away from you, you can redeem them and rescue them from a lifetime of physical, emotional, and mental destruction. Your beauty secrets are sacred no matter what has happened to them in the past. You have the right to reclaim them and find redemption moving forward. Visit your painful memories in a gentle way and grace-filled way, seeking professional help if you need it. You need to know there is hope to restore the sacredness that is you, for indeed many men and women have.

Extend inner hospitality to yourself on the path to a more positive body image. Make peace with who you are. We have a sacred duty to extend kindness towards our past and our negative traits. Everyone has qualities or thoughts in our hearts that are awkward or destructive. The more we run from them, the faster they pursue us. Accept them as a part of your humanness and choose to let them become something positive instead.

PART TWO TAKE AWAYS

There are many outside influences and personal habits or beliefs that may shape our confidence, awareness and understanding we have of our selves. Hopefully, you've begun to gain a better insight into these through what you've read here. Here are some questions to consider as you finish this section:

1. **DISTRACTIONS** What are some significant distractions in your life that might be skewing your confidence, blurring your sense of self-awareness or keeping you from finding the tools to better insight, understanding and healthy habits?

2. **DIRECTION** What direction would you like to head? More self-awareness? Better management of stress? Wisdom to make better decisions? Healthier lifestyle? Stronger faith? Write down some core goals here that you'd like to achieve or your mission statement.

3. **DECISIONS** What priorities must you re-align to reach these goals? Part II's focus is primarily on your core connections with yourself and understanding your self better. We can become better when we consciously make decisions that align with our goals. It may help to write down decisions you can make in three columns: those that align with your goals, those that do not and those that might be neutral. Keep in mind that all decisions come with a consequence, some more short term than others. It will take practice to see how some decisions may end up in one category or another depending on the time frame.

Goal	Choice	Aligns	Does not align	Neutral
Ex: Build confidence	Watch the Bachelorette		X	
	Take a pottery class			X

A Final Note On Core Connections

YOU ARE WORTH IT!

We may not always feel we deserve it. Life happens and we put self-care on the back-burner. As I write this book, I am guilty of just this. I know all the tools to caring for myself and know how important it is. In the nine months leading up to the publishing of this book I slowly said "yes" to many little things. Over the course time, I ultimately was involved in three different ministries, a multi-faceted home-based business, advocacy work and joined a networking group. By month nine I was beginning to hit the wall. The crash came one week when I missed three major appointments. I knew something had to give as well as taking in some self-care. I had known what to do as this book was begun over four years ago and practiced for many years prior, but I diminished the importance of each and every little care adding up to a big influence in my health and well-being. Don't get me wrong, these rituals in self-care are not permission to overload your schedule. Part of the process is developing the self-awareness to create safe boundaries for your physical, emotional and spiritual well-being to prevent future train wrecks. Having a healthy baseline of the self-awareness in your basic needs, your emotional state, and your spirituality will go a long way in preparing you for future challenges that don't have to end in a crash.

Why is it sometimes easier to see the value in others but not in ourselves? There is a purpose for your life! You can live with abundance, and often the biggest obstacle is our own self and understanding our healthy desires. Give yourself the love, practice receiving this gift of Self-Care as a stepping stone to complete healing of your mind, body and spirit. Nurture your Soul. Jesus said "I was hungry and you gave me something to eat, I was thirsty and you gave me something to drink, I was a stranger and you invited me in. I needed clothes and you clothed me. I was sick and you looked after me, I was in prison and you came to visit me…I tell you the truth, that whatever you did for one of the least of these, you did for me." (Matthew 25:35-40.) Yes, these are physical acts of kindness, but they involve giving and receiving, soul-connecting actions. They can be done with a loving, kind spirit. Jesus tells us that when we love others, it's like loving Him, to love our neighbors as we love ourselves. Do you love yourself? Is it easier for you to love others than it is to love yourself? For some of us it might be helpful to think of loving ourselves as we love our neighbors. He does. Deep down inside, we all desire to be better at some level. We suppress those healthy desires and it will take practice to bring them back to life. You can ignite them again with these small exercises and choices in self-care.

So let's explore your choices!

CHOICE CONNECTIONS

Lifestyle choices that take us closer to
or
Farther from healing and wellness

Every choice we make in our lives is an opportunity to build confidence, have better self-awareness and deepen our faith/understanding of our place in this world. Two Inches of Wool was written to present and/or remind you of the simple, beautiful and effective choices that are available daily to help you optimize your physical, mental and spiritual health. Yes, some of these might require a quick trip to the local farmer's market or craft shop, but many of them are simple to put together. Some of these ideas may be springboards to other creative and useful ideas over time or combined with ideas from friends. Later in the final section of this book, you will find me encouraging you to do more of these things with friends to broaden your experience and deepen your connections.

Because there are so many new ideas here, I urge you to adopt new habits one or two at a time and add a new one once you've established them. We've discussed the foundational thinking behind many of these choices in Part II, and you may want to review those principles from time to time as you explore the choices ahead. But these sections of ideas and lists are written with the intent to inspire you to find routines that will stick and be enjoyable for you. If you like what you're doing, you're more likely to keep doing it. Researchers find that it takes about three weeks to form new habits. Rather than looking at each point as a specific new habit (for example, eating more broccoli) look at them as clustered habits: going to the farmer's market or local organic market once a week to discover new foods, recipes and routines. Meet up with some friends several weeks in a row to create an art project and explore different hobbies to see what you enjoy while hanging out with others in healthy environments. Routines can help us stay on track with new habits, but sometimes too much rigidity in a lot of areas at the same time may set us up for feelings of failure if we don't meet our expectations for a day or two. Stay on track with small victories and give yourself credit for each small choice you make for the better. And by all means, share your findings with others!

A final suggestion before we begin:

Practicing delayed gratification can be a great way to build in some accountability to new choices. Choose something you'd like to trade out - for example the drive thru coffee drink you get each morning on the way to school that's filled with 30 grams of sugar. Decide how long you'd like to go without, maybe making your own healthy version at home with whole food ingredients. Put the money in a jar that you'd otherwise spend on the coffee drink and after a week celebrate in some way using that money for something else. Donate a portion to a charity, buy a small gift for a friend in need, or save it for a rainy day. When you take the focus and reward off of yourself sometimes, it can be a great encouragement to stay the course because you'll receive something more than material rewards. Transfer your physical cravings into an emotionally filled spiritual act of kindness for someone else. This is how God often uses our weakness as His strength.

Building confidence is like a growing plant. When you are rooted in healthy connections in faith, yourself and others your confidence can come from a stable, unchanging source. the trunk delivers nutrients to the branches and supports the tree in the world. This can represent all the positive choices you make that branch out into various areas and help you grow into a strong, healthy person. The leaves extend from the trees branches as growth that can bless the world around you with fruit, shade, and seeds that can be shared with others. All parts of our being were designed to operate in harmony, growing towards the same goals. Everything is connected and when your physical body, emotional well-being and faith are all aligned to make the best choices in your life you will have confidence to endure the storms of life.

Chapter 6: Be Present

AWARENESS THROUGH YOUR FIVE SENSES

Every day we are bombarded with sensory images that fill our brain's limbic system (emotional center). Our body gathers both valuable and irrelevant data at an alarming rate, and the brain instantly or in delay sorts through all of it. Being able to stop at any time and focus in on what we are sensing is an incredibly useful skill. If we don't ever pause to do this, we are missing an opportunity to process the information for decision-making and improvement.

Although all this processing begins in physical ways via our five senses, it eventually influences our thoughts and our spirit. There is mounting research showing that when we attend to our physical needs and responses, there is a healing that takes place in the brain as well. The Vagus Nerve in particular senses and reaches all our major organs, including the digestive organs (where our "gut instincts" are centered). Aside from the spinal cord, it is the largest nerve network on our body. It is constantly sending and receiving message to and from the brain with status updates. When we stop and attend to our body's needs in any given circumstance, the Vagus Nerve send signals to the brain to move out of stress, even fight/flight/freeze mode into a rest mode. Though our bodies were designed to balance themselves, there are many things that desensitize our nervous systems: overuse of prescription drugs and over-the-counter medicines, man-made chemicals in our foods, cleaners and scents, constant noise and movement. Making conscious decisions regarding our home environment is one place you can take control of what your five senses take in and how it affects your health. You can literally regain your senses by practicing the basics of pure home and body care!

Be present. The phrase can seem elusive. I regularly ask people what they think it means because the phrase is used so often in our culture. Some have trouble putting it into words, most often it results in a definition that includes having some level of concentration. Mindfulness is paying attention to our thoughts and feelings, and involves having control over your thoughts, this is true. But for the purposes of this book, I will define being present as the physical presence in the moment, mindfulness of the realities of the same moment and full awareness of our emotional response and connective-ness to the environment. Learning to be present is actively taking part in our life, but there are some common obstacles to 'tune in' with intention. There are also simple exercises to overcome them. Let's discuss obstacles before we move on to the exercises that heal.

The first obstacle I want to discuss is the issue of not being present because of trained thinking and responses of the past. People caught in fight/flight/freeze mode are often stuck reliving the past almost as if it was a loop. They may have welded some of their thoughts or reactions to past traumas or expectations, inhibiting any new connections. This is the proverbial "I feel stuck." The messages of the past are constantly jumping on to the present, causing a disconnect between what the mind dwells on versus what the current situation is presenting. Literally, the mind is not able to reach the physical body sensations and the body is not sending clear signals to the brain so there is a distortion of communication. It's not unlike a traffic signal that might be broken as lights randomly flash green after yellow, or red when you should go.

Scientists have studied this behavior and observed typical malfunctions in the emotional brain and physical body connection. Because of the faulty wiring, so to say, the mind and body are not operating at their fullest potential. The signals get crossed, perceptions are skewed which results in unexpected responses. This is why those who suffer from PTSD often have unpredictable behavior, anger outbursts or meltdowns; the mind and the body are not aligned. When experiencing severe physical or emotional trauma, the brain jumps to protection mode and disconnects from those physical and emotional sensations. Once the trauma has passed, there are therapies and practices such as art, movement (yoga) or music therapy that utilize the five senses to reconnect the wiring. There is an enormous amount of help and hope for someone wanting to learn how to connect the mind/body/spirit with feelings once again.

Living for the future is another way we hamper our abilities to be present. Striving, reaching for goals and looking at future performance can be productive unless it drives all our energy and focus for a prolonged period of time. If we are always reaching for that which is just out of reach and not fully engaging in present-day activities with our whole heart, a sort of cognitive dissonance settles in. Cognitive dissonance says, "I want to go/be there" when the reality or possibilities are not there. There are some simple exercises we can do that will help bring you into the present that allow us to visualize the future while still being able to acknowledge the here and now.

Another way we dull our senses is through self-doubt. Self-doubt creates a barrier of fear or anxiety that literally changes your physical ability to send and receive accurate data about your environment and circumstance. The voice of fear blocks the voice of truth, and distortion triggers a level of fight/flight/freeze. Doubt and negative self-talk chip away at our abilities to live in the present and truly care for ourselves, especially when we send messages to ourselves that we are not worthy. Stick to that mission statement!

Living for the present and having self-awareness of the senses is not to be confused with an unhealthy sensual gratification habit that might be fed by ego, vanity, or raw desire. Doing what feels good in the moment as the only means to enjoy the moment can quickly turn to addiction and self-destruction. A healthy approach to being present involves making decisions about what to do in the moment that are congruent with your beliefs, your purpose and your goals. Being present has a servant-mentality about it: if it serves my health or the health of those around me, it is a practice worth doing. It also allows you to experience life on a healthy and meaningful level.

Being present also has an abundance-mentality about it. It is acknowledging and being grateful for the gifts and people around us. There is a peace in this that passes understanding, honoring our Creator by respecting and showing gratitude for all the things we are given. It is trusting that whatever is or will be can be used or reconciled for good if we harvest the abundant lessons and blessings it brings about. Abundant and grateful thinking also create a less anxious canvas upon which we can paint a healthier future. And certainly, it makes the moment a piece of divine art.

A Closer Look at Our Five Senses

The five senses (and even the 6th sense of intuition) are best under-stood from real life experiences. In the years I've been teaching yoga I've seen the powerful impact the senses have in integrating the whole self. It's made my life richer, more complex and rewarding no matter what season of life I'm in. The exercises that follow will help you experience that, too.

Before we take a look at each sense and how to exercise it, let's step over and define this thing called 'the 6th sense'. I like the Shake-spearean and Greek definitions of this sense that say it is actually 5 inward senses (or wits). Though many philosophers had varying ways of describing the wits in psychology, literature and poetry, they could be loosely classified today as:

- Common wit (coined by Aristotle as sensus communis or common sense[30])

- Imagination

- Fantasy

- Estimation (a form of instinct)

- Memory

These senses or 'wits' were/are considered the foundation of intelligence. So what did the Greek philosophers and subsequent writers know about intelligence and the senses that we, in our information society, have possibly lost sight of? What is the theory behind "gut instinct?" Bessel Van Der Kolk M.D., author or The Body Keeps The Score described it well as "Our gut feelings signal what is safe, life sustaining, or threatening, even if we cannot quite explain why we feel a particular way."[31] If our gut health is out of balance, that innate instinct can be affected as well. We'll discuss this more in the section on food and digestive health.

"Common Sense is not so common anymore" ~Voltaire

As I mentioned above, there are many things in our modern culture that have assaulted our senses and at best have caused us to take things for granted and at worst have dulled them completely. We live in a chemical world that has replaced the smell of a freshly picked orange with a chemical formulated orange mist. We've replaced the spice of a real pepper from the garden with a powder spice on our tortilla chips. We no longer crave the whole food, just a mock essence of one. And in doing so, we have allowed chemicals and flavorings to please a smell or taste artificially and without all the nutritional benefits intended by our Creator.

We are also met with challenges to our sense of sight all day long.

Images of violence and sex permeate the television and print ads so much so that in 1950 when 75% of American homes had a television set, studies were already being done on how the growing violence was affecting children and adults. Television violence was what actually made violent scenes in comic books a hotter market as children were drawn to more intense levels of action (which became quite a controversy).[32] Ever since, we all can attest to the fact that the limits of sex and violence on television and in some forms of music continue to be pushed further and further. The result is a numbing of our culture to not only the acts of violence, but also the effects and outcomes.

We certainly could continue on with many more things that dull our senses such as drugs, energy stimulants, all of which more often compound problems different from ones the users are seeking to alleviate. But sometimes we even choose to use good things to numb our senses such as music. There are many children and even adults who can no longer fall asleep in silence but need to be plugged in to headphones to help them pass out. The ability to rest and let the body reset at night is even disturbed. Too much of anything is not good and moderation is the best practice in life. We can work through these exercises that follow, but they will be less than ideal if we have addictive behaviors that are skewing our perceptions. If you are suffering from any addiction, make sure you get help and support from a professional. Our five senses do work together, and if we deprive or oppress one, it will most likely affect the others. Anyone who has suffered injury in one or more of the senses may tell you that others pick up the disparity and work harder to tune-in the senses that are fully operating. That is a powerful concept to those who have no choice, but for those of us who do, the healthier choice is to nurture and care for each sense.

You'll find that no matter where you are at in life, there are simple exercises that will help awaken your body to the world around you. If you've suffered any major trauma, it's even more important to practice these exercises as they bring us into the Present. They can be practiced anytime or repeated as you like. In fact, the more often you include activities like these in a part of your everyday life, the more heightened your senses will become and the better you can move yourself into the Present. You may also find that as your 5 senses sharpen, your common sense (and wits) will improve as well. A remarkable side effect of removing substances that are dulling your physical body such as chemicals in your environment is often clearer thinking! You'll have a better sense of your priorities and your Self. Combine any of these activities with prayer and meditation and you'll have a powerful exercise of living in the Present with our mighty God.

Tuning-in to your senses is an easy way to begin putting yourself back behind the steering wheel. In a world that makes it easy to "follow" others (a benefit of technology) we have made ourselves vulnerable to losing our identity and perspective. Not all things in the moment or in virtual reality are as they appear. We need to re-awaken our senses and our sense of what makes sense (pardon the pun) or risk losing the effectiveness of our systems to guide us.

Exercising your senses will:

- Improve your self-awareness.

- Make your self-care routines more effective.

- Help you see what your priorities are.

- Expand your ability to create and imagine

- Determine where you are expending your energy.

- Recognize your responses to different situations and stimulus.

Exercising your senses will lead you to make the best choices in your life.

Sight

It's easy to think of sight as the literal function of our eyes, but our sight also involves our perception of the world around us. As we consider ways to stimulate our sense of sight, let's keep in mind the actual world we see as well as how we perceive situations, surroundings, and relationships in a more intuitive sense of sight.

Do you recall the last time you tried to look at the world through someone else eyes? My oldest sister was severely disabled and disfigured. She lived her short 25 years of life in a full-time medical facility. Those who didn't know her might have been repulsed by her physical appearance. In fact, there was one Christmas we went to visit her and found the staff had actually put her into a closed closet alone so other visitors wouldn't be disturbed by her presence in the visiting area. This is subhuman treatment, no one deserves this. How often do we put great emphasis on what we see with our eyes before lingering into a deeper understanding of a person, situation or relationship? Luann was my sister, a person with a soul. I could see past the physical into her beautiful spirit. She was fully alive inside that broken body. Our eyes would connect and I could see into her spirit as a human being with unlimited potential. I saw a person who wanted to be accepted and loved, but couldn't communicate it because her mental capacity was that of a three year old. I saw and responded to her humanity. Seeing beyond the obvious. It stirred my natural instincts to just love her. Her life made an imprint on my heart.

We can experience so much more in life if we look beyond the obvious, fight our natural instincts to allow first impressions to influence us, and keep our eyes and heart open to underlying factors in a situation that might give us a different perspective and understanding. Our lives will become richer and relationships more authentic if we awaken our sense of sight beyond the visual.

We can all take time to really see the world and the people in our lives. Stop what you're doing and just look, observe and be. Look past the obvious. Your engagement in the world will grow deeper just by noticing the small details about people and your surroundings. When we see the world as it is we become a part of it, not just spectators. Visit an art studio or museum and learn how to view what you are seeing from someone who can teach you. Next time you are at a park, relax and watch joyful children play. Look out your window and gaze a little longer until you notice something new. Easier yet, look closely at the back of your hand and notice the incredible intricacy of the landscape there! Seeing the complexity of people and our world, anything, gives us an appreciation and wonder of all things created.

Improving our "sight" is an ongoing process and can be influential in shaping confidence in ourselves, our beliefs, and developing skills in discernment. Our faith can also be impacted by what we "see". Throughout the Bible there are almost 600 references to sight.[33] In Genesis 2, God creates every tree that is pleasant to "sight".[34] Our sight is a gift that God intended for us to enjoy. There are several illustrations that speak of God "seeing" us and knowing our hearts. Many of the situations refer to our perceptions of others or God's perceptions of our heart, to have favor with Him or not. There are many people healed by Jesus, including blind men who could see again. Jesus also healed some in sight by opening their eyes in faith. Paul is one man in the Bible who had his eyes in faith blown wide open.

In his younger years, Paul was known as Saul. As Saul, he was a powerful ruler who made it his mission to kill followers of Jesus. He has a direct encounter with Jesus. Saul is with some others who did not directly "see" Jesus, but instead "saw a light". Saul is stricken completely blind in not only a literal sight sense, but also from a sense of spiritual bankruptcy. After enduring three days of blindness Jesus sends a messenger, Ananias, to Saul to tell him he is to be an instrument of God to share the Gospel with the world. Ananias puts his hands on Saul and the scales fall from his eyes so he can see again. After this he becomes baptized and eats again for strength. Through this conversion, Saul changes his name to Paul. He would go on to write 14 of the 27 books of the New Testament in the Bible because of this divine mission.[35]

Just as Paul didn't realize he was blind in a spiritual sense before meeting Jesus, we can be blind to our own perspectives. Improving your sense of sight will begin to open up new understanding in your physical body, your emotions and your spirit if you are open to receiving it.

In improving our "sight" we definitely still want to consider practical steps we can take to protect our physical eyesight. We know that our quality of sight may diminish with age, but some modern technology is accelerating those effects. You can take some intentional measures to protect your eyes. Digital electronics have put a huge stress on our eyes. Check out the section on Digital Detox for more ideas to protect your eyesight from strains on prolonged computer and phone use.

Look, gaze, study, notice, browse, peer, monitor, examine, observe, behold, distinguish and recognize! Begin with things that you enjoy and be creative. You've probably already done this subconsciously with your interests and hobbies, but step out of your "familiar zone." Even the initially "ugly" can be studied to find redeeming beauty or ideas. Notice color, shape, lighting, motion, contrast, and depth. If you find you are drawn to certain images, consider collecting them. If you find a single scene or item that moves you as you view it, bring it into your presence daily by placing it or a picture of it in a prominent place in your home.

Learning to literally SEE things anew will be a transferable skill as you learn to see events and people anew. Through the act of studying visuals and exercising different perspectives, we can be inspired to look differently at past struggles and difficult people and empower ourselves to find redeeming pieces and new insights. We will find that we now have more power and control over past influences to apply to our goals and desires ahead. See redemption, see possibilities, see new relationships, see beauty and see how all things can be made new!

"Blessed are the pure in heart for they shall see God" Matthew 5:8

Taste

The Bible tells us that God created the world and that all He created was good. We were designed with intricate senses including our taste buds that detect sweet, sour, salty, bitter and savory flavors. This construction of our senses can take on a divine view as we read, "taste and see that the Lord is good".[36] This figurative use of taste connects our literal sense of taste with good-tasting foods as we can imagine a flavor-packed relationship with someone who loves us. As we discussed above, we live in a processed, packaged, take out world where food is not what it used to be. Food additives like MSG (monosodium glutamate) and high sodium content dull our taste buds. Artificial flavorings (which are cheaper to produce than natural flavorings) are inescapable when eating packaged foods. You can improve your sense of taste simply by taking a break from packaged and take-out meals for just a week. Make time to prepare some whole foods and savor the rich colors, textures and taste that man-made foods cannot replicate. Taste and smell are closely related so as you improve your sense of smell, real foods will become more pleasing to your palate.

Sample variations of foods in a similar category. Cheeses, for example, come in a range of tastes from a mild Gouda to a strong Bleu Cheese and many varieties in between. Begin with the mildest flavors first and finish with the strongest. Give yourself time in between samples to appreciate the flavors, textures and full sensations of taste. Be prepared, you'll most likely experience some things that do not agree with you. That's ok! It's part of the discovery, we appreciate the sweet things even more when we've had a taste of the sour. Hopefully over time, we'll become more and more open to choices that widen our appreciation and palate. And again, we can apply this process to other areas of our life, teaching us to take risks and appreciate new and adventurous opportunities.

Our tongue is not only for taste, but also for speech. Words are powerful and can penetrate our hearts. They can be life-giving or hurtful. Fill your vocabulary with positive, encouraging words that will build others and yourself up. We often hear that we are what we eat, just as powerfully, we are what we speak. Extending kindness to ourselves will make it easier to offer kindness to others.

- Surround yourself with positive affirmations, quotes or scripture. Pick your favorites and write them on notes where you'll see them, use them as a screen saver on your devices, post them on the walls of your home.
- Subscribe and follow positive blogs and websites that bring out the best in you.
- Speak truth and honesty in love, choose to use words that mirror your soul and give life to others.

Touch

Our sense of touch is probably one of the easiest senses to take for granted and most underutilized by some. My college training was in Textiles and I'm a very tactile person who enjoys exploring the texture of objects. There are many creative ways you can develop your sense of touch in everyday situations. Notice the firmness of a glass or the varied texture of your sofa, the warmth of a coffee cup or the soft fur of a puppy. What does the air around you feel like? Is it soft, cool, moist or dry? A little stillness and some noticing can bring our sense of touch alive!

Invite mindfulness into your everyday routine when you really consider the ordinary. We use our hands every day and often don't realize the impact of touch unless it is taken away from injury to the nerve endings. You've probably experienced this to some degree when wearing gloves or having a band aid stuck on the end of a finger. Our sense of touch is not limited to the hands, but our whole body. Reflexology is the application of pressure to the soles of the feet in targeted areas to relieve stress. The pressure stimulates many areas in the body to increase circulation and relax. Giving and receiving a foot massage is easy and can be very sensory when done with thought and intention. The feet are filled with thousands of nerve endings related to points over your entire body – touch on the soles of the feet is powerful.

Explore your sense of touch beyond your hands, notice how your clothing feels against your skin and sensations of hot and cold. You probably have a favorite shirt or piece of clothing, maybe it's the softness of the fabric or the way it conforms comfortably to your body.

Our sense of touch can also involve various parts of our bodies and their aches and pains. Some of these we might come to tune out over time if they are ongoing in which we can become numb. If you bump into something and then ignore your body's response to the injury, you are hampering your body's natural senses. If you have come to "live with" a certain ache or pain and have never taken time to properly address it, you may be numbing a very important clue to a distress that could compound over time. Incredibly important for women is to take time to do a self-examination of breasts; knowing your body well over time will give you the powerful benefit of noticing problems early. Simply noticing these little details will improve your sensory perception of touch and heighten your awareness of yourself and the world around you.

It's not unusual for someone who has suffered from physical abuse to have a high tolerance of pain. Our bodies were wired to respond to pain situations to keep us safe. Our brain-body connection was also wired to protect the emotional brain in the case of ongoing physical trauma by shutting off sensations of touch. As trauma survivors rehabilitate, they need to re-wire the sense of touch to connect again with their emotions and healthy brain functions. You can re-awaken these pathways when you re-consider your sense of touch in everyday situations.

Observing our physical touch is important in re-wiring body sensations that might be dulled from trauma situations. How often do we go about our days without a thought of how something feels in our hand? Observe these sensations in contact with your skin and nerve endings, really consider how it feels and what your response is emotionally or physically.

Hearing

Hearing encompasses more than just listening and this is one sense I definitely have to put more effort into practicing personally. I've heard my husband talking about where a baseball game was, but completely missed what he said because I wasn't truly listening with intent to understand. If you have children, the topic of listening and being heard is always near the top of the list of "works in progress." Computers, cell phones, and instant messaging all make it easy to communicate in multiple avenues at the same time, diluting the likelihood that everyone involved is really being heard. Our sense of listening requires an active choice on our part. We've all experienced the frustration of having a conversation with someone that feels one-sided, where the other person is not hearing or understanding us. The amount of distractions we endure numbs our ability and habit to listen intently, eventually leading to lack of deep understanding and relationship. This is huge when it comes to our ability to be present with others!

One way to practice your sense of listening is to go outside, close your eyes and try to isolate individual sounds. Listen for what is near, what is far. Listen for what is loud, what is quiet. Listen for things that respond to each other. Be present. Be a spectator. Then listen to your breath and your movements as you walk around or move about on a chair. Become a participant and add to the sound by speaking, singing or some creative sound-making.

You can practice these same things by listening to music, but focus in on instrumentation, volume, phrasing, texture and lyrical art. Consider the difference between live and recorded music, for the experience is quite remarkable! Either way, you can allow what you hear to be passive sound to accompany other activities, but you can also actively enter into the music through singing, dancing, moving or even playing! I once saw a woman performing a song with sign language; if I hadn't been there to see with my eyes I would have missed her entire performance which engaged the fullness of all my senses. Active listening means more of our senses are engaged, bringing us into the present moment in a powerful way.

"True listening brings us into touch with the unsaid. You need to train the inner eye for the invisible realm where thoughts can grow, and feelings can put down their roots."[37]

While we don't watch much tv, our family does like to watch Sherlock Holmes together. One of my older kids admitted that he's watched it at college but didn't finish it. He realized how engaged he had to be to keep up with all the dialogue and the British accents to follow the story. If he turned his listening away even for a moment, he could miss a key comment that would help to fully understanding the mystery. Our sense of listening requires an active choice on our part, we must choose to listen if we want to have the intent to understand. We've all experienced the frustration of having a conversation with someone that feels one-sided, where the other person is not hearing us literally or understanding us. Relationships can become richer when we choose to "hear" someone as a form of understanding as well as actually listening to the words with intention.

When we take time to enjoy one on one conversations and really listen to others we improve our skills of hearing, raise our awareness and tune in to our intuition. Relationships become stronger when we sense one another's emotions through dialogue. We'll be less likely to misunderstand each other if we are really listening. Improving our sense of hearing can deepen relationships as it lessens misunderstandings and turns our attention to really listening to others.

Smell

Our sense of smell is powerful for so many reasons, but most pleasurable for food, flowers, and bringing back memories. However, it's often dulled by exposure to synthetic fragrance. In addition to the risks **chemical fragrance** poses to delicate hormone balance, it also confuses other body systems.[38] The more you smell chemicals, the more dulled your olfactory senses become. Steroid nasal sprays may also dull your sense of smell which in turn makes us more inclined to use additional flavorings, salt or MSG seasoned foods to stimulate our senses. If you're using nasal sprays long term, perhaps have a conversation with your doctor to see what your alternatives are. Take a break from chemicals and just go without scent for a while. When you re-introduce scent, begin with real flowers, then essential oil products, (check http://www.EWG.org for safe options) so you're not just replacing chemicals with more chemicals. Any product with the ingredient "fragrance" is just a combination of secret chemicals that will dull your sense of smell over time. Don't be surprised if foods start to taste different as your sense of smell improves. Be patient as your body awareness adjusts to new sensations.

As I mentioned, our sense of smell has powerful links with memories. You might even begin to recall elements of your past associated with certain aromas. Use these experiences to journal and create positive feedback for yourself, even if a negative memory returns. If this happens, take a few deep breaths, acknowledge the past experience, then re-center yourself in the present. Use this time to journal about any memories or images that came to mind. If you experience anything negative or have a flashback to a traumatic memory, remind yourself where you are. Use verses and quotes to reinforce truths and promises that give you hope. And by all means, create new and wonderful memories around aromas you enjoy!

To add healthy fragrance to your self-care routines:

- Skip any products with the ingredients "fragrance or parfum". Look for products with natural essential oils and flavorings.
- Add fragrance with pure, therapeutic-grade essential oils. Ideally, get your oils from a supplier who grows, harvests, distills and packages oils on location as well as testing them for complete quality control.

As you re-explore your five senses your self-awareness broadens and improves. This will spill over into every aspect of your life in clearer perceptions, understanding and memory. Enjoy the heightened awareness - the discovery of things as they really are. All this awakening might seem like a small step, but when you pay close attention to your senses, you are living in the present.

Chapter 7: Be Mindful

PICKING YOUR THINKING

What do you hope for? What do you desire? God is pretty clear about directing our desires down healthy pathways: it should be balanced with knowledge, it can inspire righteousness, it should be paired with insight and openness, and be satisfying when directed by divine will. At the core of self-care is an element of desire. What is it that ignites passion in you? We all know the routines and challenges of life can easily squelch our desire, leaving us feel helpless or empty. Or maybe for you it's been suppressed out of living a dutiful life and just doing what you are told or feel is expected of you. Perhaps being a people-pleaser has prevented you from finding what God wanted for you as a 'desire of your heart'.

> "We hide our true desire and call it maturity. Why are we so embarrassed by our desire? Why do we pretend that we're doing fine, thank you, and that we don't need a thing?" [39]
>
> ~*The Journey of Desire*, John Elderidge

If you're making choices about your time and energy based on what everyone around you is doing, you will most likely end up feeling unsatisfied and the changes will not be lasting. But when you tap into those deeper understandings of yourself you'll discover what really brings you to life. The mind is the playing field where we can practice awakening not only healthy desire, but facing the enemies of unhealthy cravings and our natural desires to belong. It can be scary facing them, but it's essential in understanding your weaknesses as well as your God-given desires. It's ok to enjoy life, to desire good things. It is true that it is not right to use those primal instincts to cave in to overindulgence or addictive behaviors just because we can. But it is equally sad to have never followed a God-given passion as well. And so, this is where the battle of the mind begins.

"Desire without knowledge is not good-how much more will hasty feet miss the way!"
Proverbs 19:2

Healthy desire is always driven by the good. Everything God created was good. When we seek after all things in reverence to His will, the outcomes will always be positive.

The power of positivity is that it strengthens our immune system, helps us live longer, recover from injuries more quickly and it's contagious! Limit your time with the people who bring out the negative in your life and fill it with those who encourage you to make choices that will bring out the best in you.

If you'd like to understand the psychology of the brain a little more, there is a great experiment that was first created in 1951 and re-created many times since with the same results. Solomon Asch conducted the first conformity experiments in social psychology to observe individual behavior in a group setting.[40] This study was ground breaking in understanding group psychology to the point that it exposed our human nature to follow the crowd even if something is blatantly wrong in our own minds. Watching the four minute Youtube of this first study may be enlightening to your perspectives in understanding yourself and how you can be pro-active in understanding the tendencies of human behaviors of others, including yourself, in a group setting.

http:// bit.ly/AschExperiment

Here are some activities that can help you discover more about your thoughts, perspectives and feelings:

At Home:

- Watch a comedy and let yourself laugh. Look for a clean-cut version like Tim Hawkins.
- Recite a scripture verse, write it down and memorize it. If you want to add some depth to this exercise, breathe in an essential oil aroma whenever you read it. After repetition, the smell of that essential oil may be imprinted on your memory along with the verse. This is a great way to work on re-programming your memories to include positive affirmations alongside our sense of smell.
- Practice mindful meditation, even 10 minutes a day is super helpful. Work on being still with focused thoughts, as you read a quote or verse. If your mind begins to wander, bring yourself back to the words and their meaning to you. Praying is also a great way to fill your meditative time.
- Write a kind letter to someone and send it in the mail. Be as specific as you can and share any thought-filled words.
- Write out 10 things you like about yourself, keep it in a place where you can see it regularly.
- Open your heart to extending forgiveness by writing a forgiveness letter. The toughest part is deciding you will forgive.
- Make the ordinary Extra-ordinary. Practice delayed gratification with little things: eating a piece of chocolate, opening a letter from a friend. It's more enjoyable when you can savor the moment rather than feel like it is just another item on your "to do list".

- Practice "re-framing" and try to think of the bright side of any situation. Positive thinking strengthens the immune system. Think of the glass half-full. A fun movie that is a great example of positive thinking is "Pollyanna". You'll be entertained by the retro setting of this, too.
- Limit your cell phone use, using speakerphone when you can to increase the distance the device is from your head and turn off your wi-fi at night. Limiting your use of electronics will keep your brain waves working in their optimal zone, keeping your thoughts clear, concentration better and mind more focused.[41]
- Take a fast from distractions of social media. Our earthly minds may be easily swayed by flashy messages, comments and shares as we are tempted to follow others down a path we might not intend to go.
- Create a dream board filled with things you enjoy, would love to do, would love to be, would love to give!

Getting Out

- Attend a live concert or play, try different styles and outlets: a classical ballet or a live improv comedy, a thought provoking monologue or a stadium-filled music production. Try something you haven't before. You might discover a new favorite.
- Go to an ice-cream shop and try all kinds of ice cream. What flavors do you really like?
- Visit an art museum and consider which types of art you like. What is it you like about them? The colors? The textures? How do they make you feel? Identify thoughts they might provoke: joy, adventure, comfort, familiarity, connection or wonder. Don't be afraid if some other artworks might trigger some uncomfortable feelings. Just observe them and receive them as part of yourself at that moment.
- Go dream building: visit a cause you want to support, drive

the vehicle you'd love to own, grab brochures of places you'd love to travel, set up interviews or coffee if you can with people you admire.

- Join a positive community of people who want to grow and dream like you.

Chapter 8: Be Connected

PRACTICING MIND-BODY EXERCISES

As we discussed earlier, our beliefs can shape the expectations we have in situations of healing, hope and wisdom for guidance in all we do. Do you believe that you will be healed? Do you believe that you will become whole again? Do you realize that you can have abundant living with a clear mind, strong body and confident spirit? Do you believe that you are not alone on this journey? These are some of the spiritual questions that address physical concerns in a big way.

In order to better understand what we believe about the mind-body connection, we have to face the truths of who we are and what we believe. In part II we focused more on core beliefs of who we are right now: how you feel about your body image, how emotionally connected you are with yourself, whether you lead your life with thoughts of abundance or scarcity and understanding the levels of safety you experience, and all the moving parts that shape those beliefs. Through the practice of yoga, stretching, and breathing we will explore opportunities to enhance physical health with emotional awareness a spiritual connection. In alignment with my core beliefs, my "Holy Yoga" practice is carried out from a distinct Christ-centered focus. If it helps, you can consider this another "style" of yoga as you would learn about the foundational teachings of other styles such as Ashtanga, Hatha or Iyengar. Holy Yoga is somewhat a blend of Hatha Yoga, which is a physical practice of yoga, and Bhakti Yoga which is a yoga of devotion. When these two forms are combined into Holy Yoga's use of postures or poses, the physical practice of yoga becomes a path to being immersed in the Holy Spirit. Many yoga disciplines seek enlightenment, a deep experience of the self. The final goal of Holy Yoga is not to seek enlightenment through self-awareness but through Christ-awareness.[42]

"You will be like a well-watered garden, like a spring whose waters never fail."
Isaiah 58:11

This next section will challenge you to understand core beliefs and choices through the practice of spiritually guided movement and movement guided spirituality. How do you address your health in terms of your faith? Use the exercises in the next two sections to cultivate the space to explore these questions. If you have no direction in your beliefs, you will have no direction in the choices you make. Spending time in quiet reflection whether it's through gentle stretching or walking out in nature, teaches us to slow down and observe our physical body, emotions, thoughts and beliefs. The better you can understand yourself, the more intentional you'll be with everyday choices you make for whole living. It isn't something that should be forced. Checking off items in each area will not magically result in feelings of wholeness. Actually inviting God into all areas of your life is where the wholeness happens. The Bible tells us that we can receive this wisdom and guidance from the Holy Spirit, an active, living force of the Triune God.

"Blessed is the man who trusts in the Lord, whose confidence is in Him. He will be like a tree planted by the water that sends out it's roots by the stream. It does not fear when heat comes; it's leaves are always green. It has no worries in a year of drought and never fails to bear fruit." Jeremiah 17:7-8

What is Yoga?

Yoga has become well known as a tool to reduce stress, improve concentration and even improve health of those suffering from PTSD. It is also being prescribed more by doctors to manage heart conditions, reduce weight and maintain physical fitness. The benefits are reaching beyond the stereotype of just helping people become flexible. For those who don't fully understand yoga, it can appear to be a mystical practice with foreign language and unknown philosophies. It may feel intimidating when we first don't understand what yoga is about, so here is a little background to give you some better insight.

Yoga by definition means being yoked. We are all yoked to something whether we realize it or not. This chapter is written from a perspective of being yoked in your physical practice of stretching and moving the body with the one true God, Jesus. If you do not practice the same faith, I encourage you to just read this from a comparison and contrast of history between some major teachings.

Yoga students are often first drawn to a teacher or style of yoga. Most yoga styles originated from teachings thousands of years ago. The actual origins are not fully confirmed. While many believe that yoga originated from the Hindu culture, the earliest records of yoga life pre-dates it by thousands of years in ancient drawings found in Indus Valley Region[43]. These ancient practices have been passed down orally from teacher to student for centuries which are reflected in modern day yoga styles. Many of these "guru's" teachings are not quite complete and concise as Jesus' teachings in the Bible. For example, Patanjali was a yoga teacher who wrote many early yogic teachings. He described "enlightenment" (a path to attaining the highest level in yoga) as the "peace that passeth all understanding." This text is complete at the point of "understanding" with no godly entity as a part of the enlightenment, it is achieved out of our own efforts. By contrast, we can read in the Bible that this peace involves an active and living God who protects and guides us:

"Do not be anxious about anything, but in everything, by prayer and petition, with thanksgiving, present your requests to God. And the peace of God, which transcends all understanding, will guard your hearts and your minds in Christ Jesus."

Philippians 4:7

Many world religions are based on the teachings of a guru or great leader: Mohammed and the Koran, Buddha and the Noble Path, Krishna and the Bhagavad Gita. Ultimately, all of these are texts written by earthly people who give their teachings of how you should live. Ravi Zacharias notes the distinction of Jesus:

"Jesus did not only teach or expound His message. He was identical with His message. "In Him," say the Scriptures, "dwelt the fullness of the Godhead bodily."[44] He did not just proclaim truth. He said, "I am the truth."[45] He did not just show a way. He said "I am the Way."[46] He did not just open up vistas. He said "I am the door."[47] "I am the Good Shepherd."[48] "I am the resurrection and the life."[49] "I am the I AM."[50]

Regardless of the history of the yoga practice, it ultimately is a very personal choice how you practice and no one can make you believe anything you do not want to believe without your permission. What does matter is that you are true to yourself and seek truth in any situation whether it's in a yoga practice, nutrition program, relationships or professional development. What matters is your heart situation and the beliefs that carry you through day to day as a whole person. If you are wrestling with your own faith or understanding what your beliefs are, may I encourage you to continue thinking about the concepts and questions in Part II.

As a health advocate with a Christ-centered world view, I can talk about other religions and philosophy in an academic way, but the wisdom and knowledge I experience and share comes from what I know to be true in my life. In restating that, some talk about the "universe" or "mother nature" as a generic entity, but it becomes unclear as to how the "universe" can know us, know us as intimately as caring God. It's unclear how we can relate to the "universe" or "mother nature" in a way that these entities will relate back. I do know that the Bible has a clear invitation to enter into a relationship with a living God who is active in our lives, our world and our eternity. It is a complete choice of free will to surrender to a relational God in this way.

For those of you grounded in faith, yoga can be a rich experience to really connect your mind, body and your spirit as you deepen your beliefs through a physical practice. I'm not sure that I would recommend a yoga class to anyone without knowing who the teacher is and where the student is on a physical, emotional and spiritual level. For obvious reasons, each class is different based on the teacher's beliefs, style and focus during class.

> "May the God of hope fill you with all joy and peace as you trust in Him, so that you may overflow with hope by the power of the Holy Spirit."
>
> Romans 15:13

That said, I've seen many arguments both for and against the practice of yoga in the space of a Christian faith. I have come to the conclusion that anything in this world has the potential to draw us closer to our creator or push us further into the worship of ourselves or idols. If we were to eliminate any potential "stumbling blocks" in our lives, we would have nothing left in the world. This chapter is written from a perspective that Christ followers have an opportunity to reclaim fullness of the mind, body and the spirit, without compromising your beliefs and values. When we practice stretching, body movement and intentional meditation, we are treating our body as a sacred place, a temple of the Holy Spirit. Practicing yoga gives us real life tools in living with intention and holding our thoughts captive in Christ. As we practice more stillness and solitude, we open our hearts to better understanding of our brokenness and begin to see a clearer path to making better choices in our thoughts, words and actions.

The modern day church does a great job of reaching the intellect and the heart, but seems to have fallen short of integrating the physical body into the fullness of our being. Modern yoga practitioners have embraced this fullness in the context of different spiritual beliefs. Are we missing an opportunity to live in the fullness of God's grace if we limit His access into the fullness of our being in any area of our life? What does it look like for you to invite God into the space of your physical body?

As Bill Hybels often speaks at the Global Leadership Summit, "we have a lot that we can learn from each other." What can the modern day church learn from some of the traditional yogic practices without feeling like we are sacrificing our faith on the altar of paganism? Does it have to be an all or nothing approach? What principles are black and white? And which are not? How do we define a right and wrong way to worship? What does it mean to live out our faith completely?

I've been in a unique position since practicing yoga, where I may be too secular for some who call themselves Christians, and too Christian for traditional yogis. While I've met many people with the same faith as mine who see the benefits of yoga, I sense that some are still afraid of it. For many, the unknown can initiate feelings of fear, but God tells us directly that fear is not from Him. Fear can come from anything we might not understand, that's why it's so important to be grounded in faith no matter how you are living. God can redeem anything for His good purpose and use any activity to bring us deeper in relationship with Him if our heart is in the right place, it is our responsibility to seek Him and our choice to receive His grace. Bryan Bishop challenges Christ followers to consider all the different ways that earthly people can worship the one True God. He states

"From the beginning to the end of the Bible, God uses the language and imagery of the heathen world to communicate with His people."

116

Throughout history, Christians have converted pagan holidays like Christmas (Saturnalia, the Roman winter solstice festival) and Easter (derived from the Latin "April" as "Eosturmonath', or 'Paschal Month') and redeemed them as a personal celebration of faith. Is yoga no different? Are we limiting our faith in the God of the Universe by thinking He cannot use even yoga to heal the soul and find the lost? During several mission trips overseas, I've heard direct stories about people having faith awakenings from the one True God without ever having any Biblical teachings or interaction with other Christ followers. I believe that God has already overcome the world and that He can work through any means to reach the heart. Are we willing to receive it in whatever form it comes? As humans, we often just see the exterior of each person, but it is in our heart that our thoughts, intentions and beliefs are formed. This is a profound truth that reveals the intention and power of God.

If you are going to practice yoga as a form of exercise, then see it as simple body movement, improving flexibility and gaining awareness of your breath. It's our heart condition and what we worship internally that sets the tone for how we live out our faith. For some, simple stillness the way to meditate on scripture. For others of us, physical movement through the form of yoga stretches and poses is an important way to not only worship our creator and meditate on His glory, but also a method to heal the emotional and spiritual parts of our being.

When I began practicing yoga I worked as a fitness instructor at a local YMCA. I had just taken my first yoga class and loved the stretching and movement that reminded me of my gymnastic's training years ago. I had no pre-conceived notions about what I was practicing and looked at it purely as exercise. This was the space I discovered stillness and began to be comfortable with the emotional side of my self. I began to reflect more and understand my own motives, feelings and beliefs. Gradually as I stretched my body through yoga, it challenged me to stretch my mind, to become more flexible in my thinking and I began to grow deeper in my faith in Jesus and who I was created to be. When I was younger, I was probably quite stubborn and narrow minded. Yoga has given me perspectives and the space to see the world in a broader sense and helped me find not only better self-awareness, but self-acceptance like I had never realized before.

Stretching, Healing and Personal Challenge

Since that traditional training, I've been fortunate to become connected with the Holy Yoga community which practices with the goal of finding better "Christ-awareness" in our own mind, body and spirit. Regardless of what your faith beliefs are, our bodies have the potential to heal and be whole through the practice of yoga. What is amazing is that scientists continue to find more evidence of the healing that occurs in our brains through the physical practice of yoga which encompasses our thoughts and emotions in the process.[51] Practicing yoga is very different physiologically than jumping on a treadmill and getting your heart rate going. The emotional and physical connections of the body and brain are becoming re-wired through a yoga practice. I hope this inspires you.

There is growing research showing the clearer connections of practicing yoga and the development of confidence and overcoming trauma, including PTSD.[52] These studies are showing significant decreases in these chronic stress symptoms including negative tension, dissociative and depressive states after consistently practicing yoga.[53][54]

Digging deeper and knowing that physical movement is so important when you feel at the end of emotional strength, there are strong foundations in yoga that will support the mind, body, spirit connection. The poses that require physical strength can be a reminder that God is our strength.[55] He shows up to carry us through even the most difficult of circumstances. Uncomfortable poses challenge us to be patient with the discomfort until we move out of it. It will happen eventually, it just takes time. Life gets pretty uncomfortable, doesn't it? Practicing difficult poses trains us to work through the discomfort, not avoid it. Real growth happens in our physical, emotional and spiritual selves when we work through the hard things. Defining what is a difficult pose is relevant to each person. One person might find that lying on the back for the resting corpse pose or "Savasana" is a trigger to traumatic events, while another person finds it restful. This is totally normal. The important step in practicing yoga is to increase your awareness of what is and is not uncomfortable and how that might be changing over time as it coincides with your thoughts, emotions and full-body awareness.

When we put ourselves in positive stress situations through yoga poses, it helps us re-program our mind and our body to stay in the present and manage the discomfort, stretch and flow of the body. When emotions are triggered from trauma or previous experiences, being present in a yoga pose can help us face those memories in a mindful, safe way. Our brain creates new pathways when we detect new sensations in our body during poses that might occur simultaneously with memories or reflections. When this happens, our first reaction may be to shut off the feeling of fear or apprehension arising from emotional or physical challenges that might make us feel unsafe. You have a choice to pull out of any posture and move into a safe place, child's pose is a good option. You have full control to stop a pose or movement at any time. If you feel safe in the observation, I encourage you to take notice and just hold on to the exploration as a pathway to re-training your brain in this new situation.

As you practice poses and open your heart to receiving God's healing, you may observe that emotions will surface. Allow yourself to feel these emotions, but keep grounded in your breath. If you feel overwhelmed in a posture, allow yourself to come out if you need to but do it without any shame or guilt. In yoga, as in our faith, there is no judgement from each of us. Invite God into your practice and allow Him to pour out His grace on you, receive His full acceptance and extend that same love, care and acceptance to yourself. Allow yourself to pull out of any pose if you feel you need the self-care, otherwise be patient as you work through any resistance in your body knowing that these responses are not unusual. Working through difficult points in a pose gives you strength physically and emotionally to handle tough challenges off your mat. It can be a spiritual practice if you choose to pray, meditate on scripture and invite God into your practice. Here are some simple yoga postures and meditations you can consider applying. You have full freedom to use other verses or uplifting quotes that you feel fit your life right now. One of the key points of yoga is to think about how you are feeling through the poses, good and bad. Use these exercises to practice observing your mind, body and spirit.

"Self-regulation involves relying on the internal-ness of your body" - Bessel Van Der Koss M.D.

A Special Note On Healthy Backs

The back is one of the places many people hold stress. It's not uncommon for a back to go out at the least convenient times (not like any time is convenient!). There was one season I threw out my lower back, my weak spot, just days before I had to film a fitness training video. I didn't do anything different than I had been the months prior, but the stress merged with a single body movement that put my back in a vulnerable position. The body remembers stress and trauma, making us vulnerable to re-injury. Practicing yoga helps us to re-program the muscles, joints, even the mind and create new pathways in the brain for a healthier outlook and physical response to the daily stressors of life. Practice these postures to strengthen your deep core muscles that hold your vertebrae in alignment and improve your posture so you are stronger in times of stress. Keep your mind and spirit engaged with each exercise and refuse to let your To-Do list invade your space.

Key Points

- Listen to your body. Stop if you feel pinching or sharpness in the back.
- Keep your core muscles engaged to protect the back muscles.
- Move slowly and methodically, no sudden moves!

Photos of Plank Pose and preparation for Half Bow Pose, kneeling.
http://bit.ly/Yoga4HealthyBacks

REFLECT/DEVOTION

Think of all the ways you have grown stronger, more aware in your mind, body and spirit. Ask God for wisdom in understanding yourself better so you can choose what is good and right and true.

JOB 29:20 (NIV) "My glory will remain fresh in me, the bow ever new in my hand". Allow God to bring you refreshment, renewal, prepared for whatever comes your way. He will strengthen you and guide you in what you need.

Beginning a Yoga Practice

MOUNTAIN POSE

1. Put your feet on solid ground. Any postures placing weight on the feet are very stabilizing.
2. Think of a tree rooted in the ground.
3. Standing postures give us stability, clearer thinking and calm as we check our posture. Standing poses can give us confidence when we don't feel it on the inside. It's really a simple pose, but can be powerful.
4. How sturdy do you feel on your feet? Being grounded is helpful as you begin to understand where your strength comes from. Sometimes it may not always seem clear.

KEY POINTS OF MOUNTAIN POSE

- Notice the weight in your feet. Your stability should be in the center of the feet. It may help to shift your feet slightly forward to the toes, then back to the heels. Settle in the middle of the feet where it's more secure.
- Tighten your thighs and tuck your tailbone in slightly.
- Draw your naval in towards your spine and open your heart, rolling the shoulders back.
- Stand tall and feel length in your spine.
- Breathe gently but intentionally.

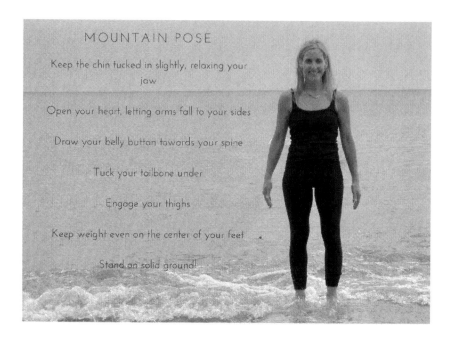

MOUNTAIN POSE

Keep the chin tucked in slightly, relaxing your jaw

Open your heart, letting arms fall to your sides

Draw your belly button towards your spine

Tuck your tailbone under

Engage your thighs

Keep weight even on the center of your feet

Stand on solid ground!

REFLECT/DEVOTION

Where does your strength come from? Standing in Mountain Pose can give you more self-awareness of where, who or what you look to for your strength. As you practice mountain pose, meditate on how consistent your source of strength is. Does it shift from day to day or is it like a rock, a sturdy clear foundation that never changes? Is your foundation an entity that you have confident assurance of how it will influence you and strengthen you day to day?

God wants to be your strength because He cares for you. I know I often take my life into my own hands because it's something I have control over, at least on the surface it might seem so. He also tells us "My grace is sufficient for you, for my power is made perfect in weakness." So now I am glad to boast about my weaknesses, so that the power of Christ can work through me. 2 Corinthians 12:9. (NIV, NLV). It's precisely those moments when we feel weakest that God shows up to carry us through. As you strengthen your legs and posture in Mountain

124

Pose, meditate on looking to your faith as a strong foundation that supports how you live out your life day to day.

Ephesians 6:10-18 talks about putting on the full armor of God to protect us emotionally and spiritually. We can add in the dimension of our physical body when we focus on the thoughts from Biblical scripture: "Finally, be strengthened in the Lord and the strength of His power. Put on the full armor of God, so that you may be able to stand your ground...stand firm, have your feet fitted with readiness that comes from the gospel of peace."

ARM STRETCHES

Elongating the muscles in the arms can extend and release tension in the chest and upper back. These muscles groups often get tense from stressed posture.

Extend your arm stretches to your hands and fingers, interlacing them and pressing the palms away from your body. This is an easy exercise to get your blood flowing if you are on a long flight or car ride (as long as you aren't the one driving!) Stretching opens up pathways in your nervous and circulatory system so your body can operate most efficiently.

KEY POINTS

- Practice several short stretches that are repeated rather than one long stretch.
- Stop the stretch if you feel any tingling or numbness in your arms.
- Focus on keeping your neck and shoulders relaxed as you extend the arms.

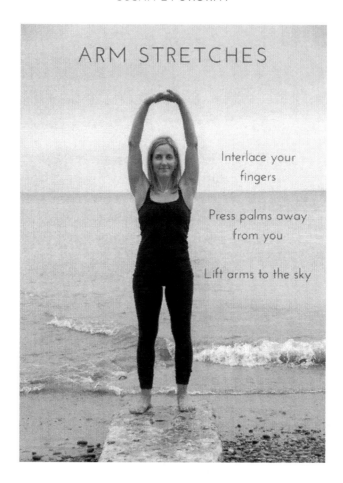

REFLECT/DEVOTION

As you reach and stretch your arms, meditate on where you strive and reach for a better path in life, to become more whole in mind, body and spirit. Meditate on what good you can bring into the world and how you can be a light in all the choices you make. Psalm 71:19 (NIV) "Your righteousness reaches to the skies, O God, you who have done great things. Who, O God, is like you?"

NECK STRETCHES

There are 21 different muscles in your neck, so take time to explore different stretches. The neck muscles are one of the most common areas our body rebels when we are overstressed. Or maybe it's that we are "carrying the weight of the world" on our shoulders. Whatever the reasons, it is a common "hot spot" of stress with all those tiny muscles interacting in the same area, interfacing with the daily stressors of life. It's the equivalent of a three-dimensional spider web made out of bungee cords. We are amazing creations with very detailed design by our creator. Scientists have discovered over 4 million active receptor points in the human body that intersect our DNA with biological functions[56], that is a fearfully and wonderfully made design! I share that to give you a glimpse into the wonder of our bodies systems. Stretching your neck can involve so much more than just simple rolling of the neck to unravel some of those tight spots. Don't be afraid to explore your body's movement in these neck stretches. When you find an area of tightness, just linger a little longer as needed, add some breaths to your stretch to try and relax those muscles as you think about how they are really feeling. Keep in mind that neck tightness may stem from the base of the skull, all the way down to the upper vertebrae between the shoulder blades. This muscle group is called the Trapezoid. If you feel tightness in the neck, the real culprit may lay in an area along this muscle.

1. First turn your head side to side as if saying no, or up and down saying "Yes" (unless you are in India where the reverse is true).
2. Next, gently roll your head through the center, but do not tip your head back, this strains the vertebrae in your neck (the C-spine). Be gentle with neck stretches and go slow.

Key Points

- Move slowly.
- Explore movement gently through both sides of your neck.
- Do not drop head backwards, this will stress your upper vertebrae.

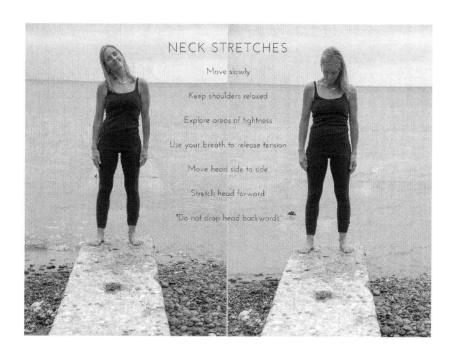

REFLECT/DEVOTIONAL

Psalm 139: 13-14 (ESV) "For you formed my inward parts; you knitted me together in my mother's womb. I praise you, for I am fearfully and wonderfully made. Wonderful are your works; my soul knows it very well." Meditate on the wonder of your body's design. You were made for good works and nothing is a surprise to your creator. there is a plan and a purpose for your life, if you want to tap into that potential to be the best you can be. Explore your neck stretches and the amazing structure of it's design and release your worries to Jesus who extends the invitation to carry the burdens in your life. In Matthew 11:29 He tells us to "Take my yoke upon you and learn from me, for I am gentle and humble in heart and you will find rest for your souls." (NIV)

FORWARD FOLD

Rolling forward and and gently stretching will relax the body, stretch muscles along the back of the legs (hamstrings) and the back, massaging the digestive organs to encourage the release of waste. You can do these simply by reaching for your feet.

1. Make sure your knees are not locked out, you can even bend your knees slightly as this takes pressure off of your back.
2. Use a towel or strap if you need - we defeat the purpose of stretching if we tense up our arms reaching for our toes! Using a strap when you first begin takes tension out of the upper body and let's us focus where we want. These folds also stretch out the back of the legs, hamstrings, as well as your back.
3. When you first practice doing forward folds, you might feel stretching in either place, maybe even in your arms as you reach. This is part of the discovery, learning more about your body and where your weaknesses and strengths lie. Embrace your body's movement no matter where you are. Look at it as discovery so you can work on relaxing the areas that are tight and strengthening the areas that are weak.

KEY POINTS

- Keep your knees soft, don't lock out the knee joints.
- Notice if you are feeling the stretch more in the back or the front of the legs. Either is fine, just noticing where the stretch is happening will bring you better awareness of your tight areas.
- Bring your feet apart to create a more gentle stretch. The

closer your feet are together the more challenging the stretch will be.

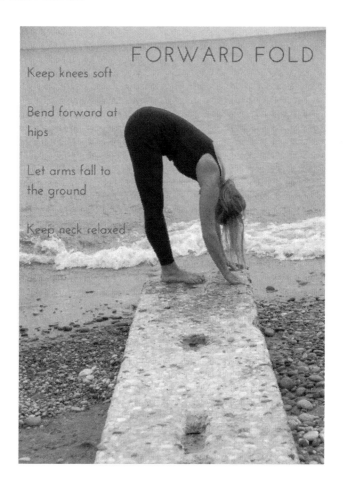

REFLECT/DEVOTIONAL

Psalm 95:6 "Come let us worship and bow down, let us kneel before our God and our creator" Meditate on how you can worship God with your body as a temple of the Holy Spirit. Think of ways that you can honor your body as a holy and sacred place to live your life. Ask God to open your eyes to anything that might keep you from receiving His wisdom, grace and favor.

TREE POSE

1. Begin standing in Mountain Pose with your arms at your sides. Balance on both feet and feel the ground evenly.
2. Shift your weight to one foot and bend the opposite knee. Reach down and draw that foot alongside your inner calf, then up the inner thigh if you have the flexibility. Do not press your foot against your knee.
3. Focus your sight on something in front of you to concentrate and stay balanced.
4. Switch legs and repeat.

Key Points of Tree Pose

- Many circumstances affect our physical balance: sleep quality, sinus congestion, injuries or surgeries to the lower limbs, core strength, back strength, emotional stress.
- Each day your balance poses may shift, but over time and with practice you can become stronger.
- Notice how your body shifts in small ways to maintain the balance.
- Focus on an object to develop better concentration.
- The height of your leg can vary, from placement on the ankle up to the inner thigh.
- Avoid pressing your foot on the knee joint.

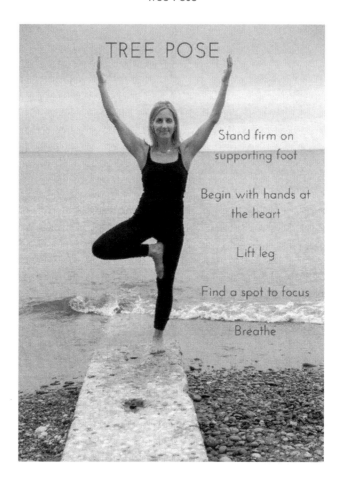

REFLECT/DEVOTIONAL

Where do you feel balanced today? Where do you feel out of balance? What is your foundation for strength, confidence and wisdom? Meditate on these thoughts as you practice Tree Pose. As your body shifts, consider all the ways you can adjust in your life to stay in balance. Rigidity in our perspectives, trying to take control over every aspect in our lives will set us up for breaking or losing balance when we least expect it. Sometimes the harder we work to control that balance the more difficult it is.

if you surrender the rhythms of your life to God our creator, He will strengthen you, keep your life in balance and guide you in all you do. "Blessed is the man who trusts in the Lord, whose trust is in the Lord. He is like a tree planted by water, that sends out it's roots by the stream, and does not fear when heat comes, for it's leaves remain green, and is not anxious in the year of drought, for it does not cease to bear fruit." Jeremiah 17: 7-8

TWISTING POSES

Twisting helps to cleanse the digestive tract and build flexibility in the spine. You can approach twisting poses in a seated position, standing or lying down.

- Turn your body to the right side first, then to the left.
- Puts gentle pressure on your digestive organs in the direction they naturally flow.
- Be aware, twisting poses may stimulate some movement in your belly!

Key Points

- Move slowly and notice the difference between sides.
- Repeat movements a few times from side to side to begin relaxing your body.
- Keep your posture tall and avoid slouching as you twist.

REFLECT/DEVOTION

Look at an area of your life that you would like to improve, change a habit or break away a negative influence. Consider this thought with intention in taking action to eliminate a bad behavior or change direction to a better way. Give yourself grace and time to reach this small goal as you face the truth in your life to walk ahead with clear thinking.

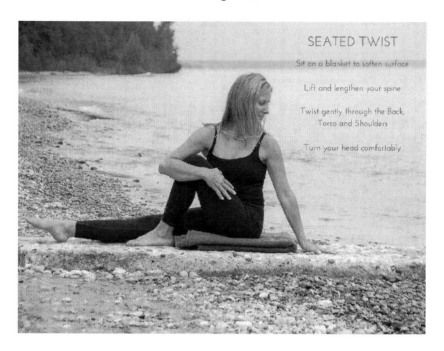

SEATED TWIST

Sit on a blanket to soften surface

Lift and lengthen your spine

Twist gently through the Back,
Torso and Shoulders

Turn your head comfortably

"With promises like this to pull us on, dear friends, let's make a clean break with everything that defiles or distracts us, both within and without. Let's make our entire lives fit and holy temples for the worship of God."
1 Corinthians 7:1 The Message

CHILD'S POSE

1. Kneel on the ground and put your head down onto your arms.
2. If you can get your forehead to the floor or onto a folded towel this slight pressure above the eyes helps calm the nervous system.
3. Place a blanket or rolled up towel under your feet, behind the knees or under your arms as needed for extra support.
4. Observe your body and what you are feeling physically, emotionally, spiritually. Don't rush.

KEY POINTS

- Desk version: sitting comfortably in your chair, rest your forehead on your forearms for 5-10 minutes.
- The goal is to find a comfortable position where you can relax your physical body.
- Focus on your breath patterns as you rest in this posture.
- Be patient and give yourself time to settle into this posture the first several times you try it to find good support for your limbs.
- This is often a calming pose, but don't be surprised if emotions begin to surface. If you are not used to being still in a mindful way, unexpected emotions may begin to bubble up. It's ok. Embrace the feelings and the thoughts with no judgement on yourself. Focus on a favorite verse or say a prayer.

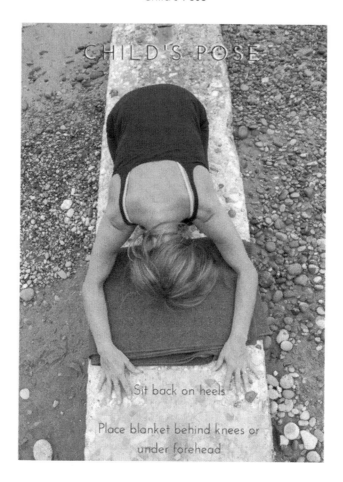

REFLECT/DEVOTION

Do you find it easy to look at life with childlike innocence, or do you tend to take on the worries of the world? If you do lean towards worrying or stressing out about earthly matters, how do you let go of those concerns to bring yourself into a place of rest? Child's Pose is a place where you can think about being a child. What is a favorite memory you have as a child? Keep this in mind, the carefree spirit of a child just being. No worries, concerns or agendas. Living freely with pure joy.

Jesus said let the little children come to me and do not hinder them. He also promoted the importance of protecting children from any harm: emotional, physical, or spiritual. As adults, it can be easy to become "stuck" in worries of the world or hold onto past hurts and trauma. Jesus invites us to come to Him as a little child and release all the weight of difficulties we might be carrying. Resting in Child's Pose can be calming to your physical body and also in your spirit as you release any heaviness in your life. Jesus invites us to give our burdens to Him so that He can carry them in exchange for His load he gives to us which is light.

LEGS EXTENDED UP THE WALL

1. Lay on the ground with your legs up the wall. This will increase blood flow and reduce fluid build up in your legs and feet.[57] This biggest challenge for some will be getting into this pose, but once you try it it's amazing! If you'd like, you can rest in this posture during a few minutes of relaxation.

2. Be still for 10 minutes. Play soothing music or enjoy the quiet. For most effectiveness, do this without interruption. No electronics, no talking, just stillness. If your mind begins to wander or think about your to do list, focus on your breath, listen for sounds around you and just notice your body and environment.

- **R**emove distractions you can: cell phone, pets, turn off tv and lights.
- **E**mbrace the present. If past or future thoughts enter in, allow yourself to observe these for a minute and then try to re-focus on something in the present moment: the temperature of the room, how your body feels supported on the floor or shifting yourself into a slightly different position.
- **S**tretch your body if you'd like, just reaching arms overhead for simple movement if you become uncomfortable with the stillness.

- **T**each yourself awareness of your thoughts, emotions, body and spirit in these moments of quiet.

REFLECT/DEVOTION

Our lives can get so busy, even when we don't have activities going on, technology makes it possible to drive our stress levels up. In what area of your life could you use more rest? Work intensity, family obligations, volunteering, extra-curricular activities? Too much of a good thing can create stress as well. Pruning away the excess in our lives can give us the margins to manage the responsibilities of life in a more effective, life-giving way. Carving out a few minutes of rest each day will go a long way to restoring yourself on a daily basis as part of a regular routine. Even if your schedule is full, you can choose to carry on your responsibilities with a restful attitude as you focus on the glass being half full. Bring gratitude with you into your busy schedule and re-focus the busy-ness into a perspective of privilege and honor. We have the energy to carry out these duties, we have a family to care for, we have a car to take us where we need to go, we get to _____, (what would you fill in the blank?).

Your spirit was designed with rest in mind to restore you. Rest is so important to God that He included it into the Ten Commandments. He even rested on the seventh day after creating the world and calls us to honor our body's with rest each week. Look at practical ways you can build in rest to each day on physical, emotional and spiritual levels. Physically, as you allow your body the rest it needs rather than pushing it beyond it's limits with artificial stimulants such as caffeine. Emotionally we can rest our body when we build in time each day for reflection, journaling and healthy communication with those in our lives. Spiritually we can rest when we meditate with intention on faith-filled verses and spending time in prayer. In the book of Mark, Jesus and His disciples are teaching thousands of people and He invites them to take rest saying "Come away by yourselves to a secluded place and rest a while" for there were many people coming and going, and they did not even have time to eat.[58] Have you ever felt so busy you didn't have time to eat? Jesus understands this and He invites us at just these moments to rest. Rest for 10 minutes to renew your perspectives, your spirit and your energy.

DISTRESS TOLERANCE

As you begin practicing yoga, you'll often find a pose that seems awkward or uncomfortable at first. It could be any pose. Keep in mind what makes one uncomfortable can vary from person to person. There is a difference between healthy risk (stretching your body a little further) and injury (taking a pose too far where you are entering an unsafe risk zone). You should never feel pain, sharpness or sudden pulls in your body. If you begin to feel too uncomfortable, you must be the one to bring yourself out of a pose. This can be challenging if you are in a class and not confident in reading your body's cues. Quiet and stillness in a yoga class gives us the opportunities to observe how we are feeling physically, emotionally, and spiritually. All these parts of our being are fully connected. Self-care is bringing yourself out of any pose whenever you need to for any reason: physical discomfort, emotional awareness or spiritual reverence.

KEY POINTS

- Extend grace to yourself and pull out of a pose if you need to for safety.
- Challenge yourself if you feel confident and secure to reach a little further or longer.
- Observe yourself physically, emotionally, spiritually in your poses and movement.

REFLECT/DEVOTION

Sometimes the greatest growth in our lives comes through moments of discomfort, those experiences that stretch us out of our comfort zone if we allow God to give us insight and wisdom. Our body speaks to us if we take the time to listen. Observe yourself in various poses and notice where you are feeling discomfort. Extending ourselves in poses will most likely cause some discomfort. If you feel this, face it straight on with courage or pull back into self-care if needed. Notice why you are feeling uncomfortable, is it physical, emotional or spiritual. Journal your thoughts afterwards if you can. Record the pose and any significance that came in your body, emotions or spirit.

In the book of Psalms in particular, God reveals the support He gives to those who trust in Him. We are never alone, He will always be beside us in everything we experience, good and bad, if we invite Him into our lives. He can be our fortress, our shelter, our counselor and even friend. Psalm 143:8-10 (NIV) "Let the morning bring me word of your unfailing love, for I have put my trust in you. Show me the way I should go, for to you I lift up my soul. Rescue me from my enemies, O Lord, for I hide myself in you. Teach me to do your will, for you are my God; may your good Spirit lead me on level ground."[59]

Breath is Life

Breath is an important tool for bringing perspectives to our thoughts, calming our emotions and connecting our body to our spirit. Because it is closely connected to our autonomic brain function, it is critical to life. As we discussed earlier it delivers fresh oxygen everywhere, enhancing all of our body functions. Breath regulation is closely tied with building resilience and recovering from trauma, partly because it helps us create new thought patterns, but also because it supports healthy brain-body physiology that affects all of our body systems. More importantly, practicing regular breath patterns helps move the body out of fight/flight/freeze mode so it can return to a calmer state. Breath has a direct impact on our Heart Rate Variability (our heart's ability to regulate itself day to day and recover from stressful situations) and the Vagus Nerve, which reaches many of our body's organs.[60] Breath work is so critical to recovery from trauma that many healing centers have programs that involve breathing exercises as part of treatment and rehabilitation. Even though breathing is so important to life, it's an area that we often freeze up in moments of stress. Many people aren't maximizing their lung capacity on a day to day basis. Here are some simple exercises for getting the most out of your breath:

1. **Breathe deeply**. Breathing delivers fresh oxygen to your body helping all systems do their job. Inhale with intention, exhale any negative thoughts. Inhale the truth, Exhale whatever is not. Add arm flow if you'd like to accentuate the breath pattern. Inhale arms rise overhead, exhale arms lower. Repeat as needed! There are many different breath patterns that can be covered in a full class. Just being aware of your breath and doing it intentionally for 3-5 minutes throughout the day can be a powerful exercise physically, emotionally and spiritually.

Calming breaths = Greater exhale than your inhale

Energizing breaths = Greater Inhale, smaller exhale

2. **Count Your Breath**: as you inhale, count to 4. As you exhale, count to 4. Gradually increase your count to maximize your breath.

3. **Check your posture.** When you are slouched down, whether sitting on the couch or driving in your car, it restricts your lung

capacity. Sit tall, lengthen your spine and breathe deeply into your fullest expansion.

4. **Formula for inhale vs exhale.**

- Calming Breaths = Greater exhale (6 counts) than your inhale (4)
- Energizing Breaths = Greater inhale (6 counts) than your exhale (4)

KEY POINTS

- Work to keep your breathing regular.
- If you feel your mind wandering as you meditate, bring your awareness back to your breath and focus on a scripture verse or a positive thought.
- Avoid holding your breath and take notice of your breath patterns throughout the day.

REFLECT/DEVOTION

Breath can give us space in our lives to not only observe our physical body, emotions and spirit, it gives us time to pause. Observe situations where you're mindful of your breath - outside or in a more relaxed state when you take intentional breaths. Notice situations where you might hold your breath: anticipation of pain (before getting a shot, going into a stressful meeting), moments of concentration or stress (driving in an unfamiliar territory, literally or figuratively) or predictable encounters that might create unsettling feelings with a person or experience. Once you notice these moments, think of intentionally breathing in and exhaling to work through any discomfort and allow your body to work through the stress in a healthy way. Proverbs 20:27 (YLT) "The breath of man is a lamp of God, searching all the inner parts of the heart"

Further Reading on Mind-Body Exercises and Rest

Holy Yoga, Brook Boon

The Healing Power of the Breath, Richard P. Brown MD

The Key Poses of Yoga, Volumes 1 & 2, Ray Long MD

Eat This Book, Eugene H. Peterson

Chapter 9: Be Creative & Playful

A BEAUTY-INSPIRED SPIRIT

"We are God's workmanship created in Christ Jesus to do good
works, which God prepared in advance for us to do."
Ephesians 2:10

Creativity is just as much about the process as it is the end result.
I've made many projects that began as an inspiration only to turn
out a mess. "THAT is not at all what I envisioned!" Not everything
goes as planned and not everything arrives at it's intended destination. But don't you love the process?! I've also created things that
turned out really cool, but the "wonderful creative process" was
closer to birth pain and labor because I put pressure on myself to
make it perfect. Our lives can be a messy work of art in progress,
and our "frame" of mind in the mess makes all the difference
between living with clenched fists or potter's hands. Clenched-fist
scarcity is thinking there are not enough art supplies to go around,
the things that make our lives a masterpiece - our experiences,
friends, relationships, recognition, confidence, acceptance, happiness. In the Bible, the word "masterpiece" has also been described
as "workmanship" a piece that has taken time and effort to create. It
is derived from the Greek word poiēma which literally translates to

"fabric". All these components of our life can be woven together into a beautiful tapestry of fabric when each is aligned with our authentic self and we live with open hands.

The creative-potter abundance is realizing I don't have to take those "materials" from others to receive them myself. There are enough "art supplies" to go around for all of us. If we add to each other's color palette the world will be a more beautiful place. Celebrate your canvas and marvel as the years go by of the masterpiece it is. We are all an amazing work in progress and we can add color to other people's masterpiece when we are encouraging with kind words and actions. Explore different activities to see what you enjoy. As you create and discover, consider how you're growing and changing in your mind, body and spirit. Invite mindfulness into your creative projects and accept yourself in this present moment as a culmination of past experiences - good and bad -that have combined into a beautiful creative mess. Creative activities give us the opportunity to observe our feelings, experiences, spirituality, in a safe space. Just remember to clean up when you are done. :)

BE CREATIVE

- Grow a seed or observe a plant that is awakening up in the Spring.Watch each day as it grows taller, stronger and be reminded of God's love for you and your life. He is the one who can till the soil of brokenness and create the perfect place for new life to grow into the fullness of His love. Hosea 10:12 "Sow for yourselves righteousness, reap the fruit of unfailing love, and break up your unplowed ground; for it is time to seek the Lord, until He comes and showers righteousness on you." Hosea 10:12
- Craft a journal and use it.
- Color one of the many new art books for grown-ups. Notice your choice of colors and how it might coincide with your emotions and spirit. Are you leaning towards bright colors or earth tones? Just observe the connection between your emotions, colors and patterns you might

make. There's no right or wrong in this, just observing the connections in your life.

- Doodle! Start small and make it grow all in the same day or add to it over time....watching it grow and shift and change, just like we are made up of micro-experiences. Some we have control over, others we don't. But we do have the choice to make any experience a beautiful outcome.

- Tear paper: make a collage out of recycle papers or magazines, cut out affirming words, glue it back onto another piece of paper, explore. Make it an activity to let go of something painful, write about it then crumple it and throw it away or toss in the campfire.

- Write a list of your gifts & attributes: something affirming, place it where you'll be reminded of it. If you don't like your handwriting, type it up on your computer with a fun font and print it out.

- Write down a list of your dreams or make a bucket list and begin to check things off. Nothing is too small to include in this list. Feeling a sense of accomplishment, even for little things, can tie us encouragement and hope on those days we need it.

- Lift someone else up by making a phone call, visiting someone homebound, sending a hand-written letter to someone on your heart and mail it. Make it personal, make it real. Not a text, email or social media post. A simple connection as a touchable memory. Let down your personal inhibitions and just focus on them and how you can encourage others.

- Paint something. Use beautiful acrylics on a canvas or dollar store watercolor paints on a piece of paper towel. Notice how the colors mix, change, and move together.

- Engage in music: Sing in the shower, dance in the rain, or just play your favorite uplifting song over and over.

- Watch a live concert, play or performance. We can watch events on youtube or the tv, but when you attend something live, it engages more of your senses. Notice all the sights, sounds, smells, textures and tastes of what you are experiencing and what emotions or thoughts it might bring on before, during and after.

- Write down a Blessed List: all the people and situations in your life you're thankful for. One at a time begin to let them know how they have impacted your life.
- Take an art class or paint with friends at a paint bar. Be your best critic and enjoy the work you created. If it's a canvas and it doesn't turn out how you planned, you can always re-purpose it and paint right over it! If it is a dark color, you can paint a layer of "Gesso" to lighten it up and prepare it for another try.
- Draw a picture of your Safe Place. Imagine a place that brings happy memories to mind. It could be something from your childhood or a place you visited. Imagine all the aspects of this place, the sights, smells, sounds, textures, tastes. Fully immerse yourself in this safe place, even invite Jesus in if you'd like. Remember what you see and draw or paint it as best as you can.
- Be creative with your food as a medium. Modern Japanese culture makes beautiful art with food in special containers called Bento Boxes (http://www.lunchbots.com/gallery/) (http://nomnompaleo.com/post/59118514268/paleo-lunchbox-roundup)
- Color the sidewalk with chalk on a sunny day. Add a wet paint brush and notice how the water changes the chalk. Observing changes in the world around us gives us practice for the times we are observing ourselves.
- Jump in puddles on a rainy day, raincoat and umbrella or barefoot in your swimming suit. (Disclaimer: not during a lightning storm!)
- Play with clay. Physically squishing clay is relaxing and therapeutic in and of itself. Add in scripture or prayer of your continued growth in faith for an activity in meditation in the present moment.

- Daydream: look at the clouds, lose yourself in a piece of art at a studio or watch a waterfall.
- Learn to sew, knit, or crochet. Take a class at a local shop or from a friend and take time to really connect with whoever is teaching you.
- Create a new hairstyle or braid someone's hair. Hair styling can be a very nurturing activity for yourself or someone special to you.

Being Playful

Does play come easy or hard for you? How did your parents influence your play as a child? Was there sibling rivalry? Were you raised in a home that was competitive or passive? How do you like to play?

My husband has observed that there were many time in my life I was either running ragged at 120 miles per hour, or crashed. Wiped out for days at a time. It's taken time, but play is one way I've found a gentle middle ground. It hasn't been easy, I admit. Being a mother of six keeps me busy. If play doesn't come easy, start with something more low key like coloring, just swinging on a swing, or trying different hobbies. The point is to just jump in and do something spontaneous and lighthearted, don't overthink it. Play helps to nourish your spirit by giving you permission to experience happiness at a simple level. Laughter actually boosts your immune system, so stick with it long enough to let down and let go. It also gives you practice in choosing activities that have a low level of responsibility or seriousness (something us serious moms could really use). There is also a low risk of failure when you choose to play and discover. We could all use more laughter, right?

The activities below might be seeds of inspiration for other areas of your life. When you open up your heart and mind to play, it often spills over into your life in unexpected, joyful ways.

- Learn some children's jokes and laugh with kids; make a habit of looking up a few good jokes each week to make laughing together an on-going memory.

- Build a fort with blankets.
- Sleep under the stars in summer with some friends and family.
- Run through a sprinkler; surprises someone with a squirt from the garden hose, or throw water balloons.
- Lay on your back and watch clouds with someone, sharing what each one looks like.
- Throw a ball, or join a recreational sports team if it fits with the family schedule.
- Go ice skating in summer at an indoor arena
- Go to a movie theater in your pajamas with friends.
- Play card games with your family or a grandparent. Keep it a simple game of war, or move into strategic games like Rummy. Have a few healthy snacks at each corner of the table.
- Have a pillow fight with your husband or kids…or all of the family!
- Blow bubbles
- Teach your dog or cat a new trick. Good luck with the cat.
- Color with crayons, or melt crayons into new shapes with pans from a resale shops.
- Draw a picture with pastels or colored pencils. Visit an art shop and learn about different techniques for creating art
- Play or learn to play a musical instrument. Ask a friend who is a musician to help you find one that will be successful for you.
- Collect something. Collecting is all about discovering beauty in everyday objects and your perceptions of them. Learn what you can about it, research on the internet or get books from a local library. Make it as simple as you'd like: different shells at the beach for an afternoon, or an ongoing collection that you research when you have the time. Take a subject like rocks. You could collect them wherever you visit, researching Geology, visiting different Geological formations like the Badlands, Grand Canyon or Utah parks and learning about their scientific properties.

Or you could just enjoy the beauty of different gemstones as you learn jewelry-making, selecting different stones for their color, texture or design.

- Learn origami and collect papers for different folding sessions.
- Explore beads and charms to make bracelets for children, friends or family. Learn different braiding techniques to make "friendship" bracelets and bring one to someone homebound or in the hospital to brighten their day.
- Piece together a large puzzle with a friend or child who you'd love to talk to more.
- Gather some friends for a roller skating party. Some rinks have decade-themed music for all ages.

Chapter 10: Be Nourishing

FEED YOUR BODY AND SOUL

"…so whether you eat or drink or whatever you do, do it all for the glory of God."
1 Corinthians 10:31

Man has a relationship with food unlike any other creature on earth. Food is often the center of social gatherings in most cultures. This evolution of food as the center of attention has morphed into a form of entertainment: food as a spectacle. At the time I was editing this book, Oreo brand announced the release of firework Oreos, which contained pop-rock type candies in the frosting layer for a flavor burst. Sure sounds fun, but there is serious concern for the ingredients! If you are going to look at food as entertainment, why not make it healthy and creative? Look at all the beautiful colors and flavors in the plants, legumes, seeds and grains. There are endless ways to nourish our senses without any laboratory-made ingredients. If we made preparation of food a skill we invested in and enjoyed, we as a culture would probably eat less and enjoy it more.

I often crave simple lingering meals with just fellowship and the nourishing of bodies. From time to time, it may be frozen or take-out pizza that fits the need. The problem creeps in when the frozen this or take out that becomes the norm and meals are a centered on a revolving door. Our family has experienced too much of that. It's all about balance, right? It can help to keep the 80/20 rule in mind when planning your meals. Eat good whole foods 80% of the time to account for the 20% when you don't have control over the meal planning or want to make an exception for special occasions. Following this rough guideline can protect you from allowing processed foods from entering too much of your diet.

Although eating is essential, it can also one of our biggest temptations. Keeping God at the center of our daily routines can keep healthy habits strong. Food is a gift from our Creator, and like all things, He asks us to be good stewards and wise consumers. We need to have a healthy relationship with food as God intended. Our responsibility is to nourish our bodies as a temple of the Holy Spirit, not use it as a crutch for a broken spirit or stuff it full of unworthy products. Everyone succumbs to emotional eating sometime or another. Lying back with a tub of ice cream or a few glasses of wine instead of dealing with an issue at hand may appear to help short term, but when it becomes the go-to habit, it could be time for some honest reflection. I've been there, done that, and left with the over-indulging stomach-ache t-shirt. And afterward, I still ended up having to deal with whatever issue I was avoiding emotionally or relationally to begin with.

For those who frequently eat to relieve stress, it is so important that you identify when you're moving towards harmful habits and stop yourself from heading down that destructive path. It's easier if you break it down to simple choices: if you're feeling that emotional pull, don't grab a valentine box of chocolate pieces or large bag of chips. Maybe consider not letting that in the house if it is too much of a temptation. You will only eat what you have in the fridge or the cupboard. If you really need to satisfy that emotional knot, you can just as easily reach for some dark chocolate and a hand full of raw almonds stashed in a jar that also has some of your favorite scriptures listed on a note. Take time to just sit and nibble while you journal, pray or call a trusted friend. The urges to over-indulge are telling you something: What are you feeling when you reach for the food or drink?

Name it.

Write it down.

Acknowledge it.

Make a plan to deal with it in a way that honors God and coincides with your core values.

In addition to being aware of our emotions at any time we're eating, the "raw materials" of nourishing our physical body comes from food. One of the most impactful effects you can have on your health is to bring as many whole foods into your diet as you can. Modern research has proven time and again the importance of eating nourishing foods to support health and wellness, but some of the first evidence is actually recorded in ancient history.

In the Bible there is an account of a man, Daniel, who falls into favor with King Nebuchadnezzar, the ruler of Babylon from 605 BC until approximately 562 BC[61] Daniel and and three of his friends are chosen to serve the in king's army and prepared to endure rigorous training alongside many other young men in preparation for servitude to the king. The young recruits were specifically selected for their intellect, wisdom and stature. During their three year training they would receive a ration of the king's choice wines and rich foods. Daniel makes a request that he and his friends refrain from eating the indulgent meals. The king's commissioner worries that the fasting on vegetables and water will deplete them of their potential and make him look like a poor commander if he has some recruits fail in their training. Daniel convinces the commissioner to approve a test for ten days so he can assess how Daniel and his friends compare to the rest of the trainees who are eating according to the king's wishes. After ten days the king's servant sees that Daniel and his friends are indeed much healthier than those who were eating the king's rich foods and they continued their diet of vegetables and water the remainder of their training.

Thousands of years ago, wine and rich foods were only fit for a king, but in our modern culture it's more convenient to eat these indulgent foods than to grow our own food or prepare home cooked meals. Fad diets will only result in temporary changes that only train our habits for a short period of time. If you want to make lasting change like Daniel did, begin to trade out a few foods at a time for a healthier, whole food option. Here are some lists of nutritious foods that are filled with nourishing goodness. When you choose nutrient-dense foods you'll get the most impact on your health, improved immune function.

So what should all this eating and preparing include? I'm glad you asked!

Essential Nutrients to Include:

- Foods that lower cortisol, one of our body's main stress hormones[62]: healthy fats, Omega 3 fats, avocados, chia seeds, extra virgin olive oil, flax, nuts, salmon.
- Vitamin C-rich veggies & fruits help repair stressed cells: raw bell peppers, broccoli, raw green cabbage, citrus fruits, dark chocolate. Eating sources of Vitamin C with iron also increases the body's absorption of the iron[63], so have a glass of orange juice with your steak or iron supplement to make the most of it's uptake into your body.
- Vitamin D boosts mood and promotes healthy brain function: eggs, mushrooms, salmon and fortified orange juices and milk.
- Super foods for brain health: healthy fats, eggs, sunflower seeds, blueberries, almonds, kale, broccoli.
- Brain Foods: nuts, seeds, leafy greens, healthy fats: avocado, salmon, ghee, olive and coconut oil.
- Serotonin is a neurotransmitter in the body, often

associated with promoting a sense of well-being and happiness in our body. Foods that are combined with a carbohydrate (oatmeal, potato, rice), encourage the natural production of Serotonin: almonds, avocado, bananas, fresh cherries, dark chocolate (70% cacao), organic eggs, leafy greens, pineapple, wild caught salmon.[64] Good combinations would be eggs and potatoes, salmon and wild rice, oatmeal and walnuts.

- B-vitamins help our brains deal with stress. They have shown to restore endorphin function and regenerate nerves making you less impulsive. Keep your diet rich in B-vitamin foods and you'll be less likely to reach for harmful foods or substances to deal with negative feelings or pain.[65] B-rich foods include nuts (especially walnuts and almonds), seeds, beans, eggs, avocados.

- Magnesium helps calm our minds, assists the body in removing toxins. Good sources include wolfberries,[66] pumpkin seeds, sunflower seeds, almonds, cashews and mung beans. Magnesium supplements have show to reduce insomnia and decrease cortisol levels in the body.[67]

- Tryptophan is a great nutrient that encourages the production of melatonin. It can be found in: bananas, cheeses, dates, nut butters, pineapple, seeds, turkey, whole grain crackers.[68]

- Eat raw fruits and vegetables for cleansing. The enzymes in raw produce help to break down foods. While it's debated at exactly what temperature, heating foods at high temps de-activates these enzymes.

- Munch on some fresh parsley or mint to freshen your breath and cleanse your system.

- Cooked veggies are more nourishing to a stressed digestive tract, just don't over-cook them or they lose all their nutrients. Some veggies should always be eaten cooked, steamed or fermented (kale, broccoli, cabbage).

- Eat organic produce when you can as they often have higher nutrient content, especially vitamin C, iron, magnesium and phosphorus. You'll also lessen your exposure to pesticides and synthetic fertilizers.[69]

- Eat organic butter and grass-fed beef when possible. Fatty tissues absorb pesticide residues and hormones during the production of animal products making their way into those end products of butter and meats. Eating these foods organically made lessens your exposure to unwanted agents.
- Clean 15: after high power washing the most common foods that are OK to eat conventionally grown because they have little or no pesticide residue, includes: onions, avocados, pineapple, mango, sweet peas, asparagus, kiwi, cabbage, eggplant, cantaloupe, watermelon, papayas, cauliflower, grapefruit, broccoli.
- Choose safe fish to eat. www.seafoodwatch.org gives up to date information on the best choices. Generally, larger fish like tuna and mahi mahi may have higher heavy metal content because they have a longer life of accumulation. Wild-caught Pacific Salmon is an excellent fish that contains good fats.
- Get your greens: leafy greens are packed with vitamin A, C and K plus many bind to heavy metals and help move them out of your body. Cilantro binds to mercury,[70] alfalfa and kelp (seaweed) have been found to bind to lead and mercury. Toss a tablespoon onto your salad, soup or sandwich for a boost of nutrients. Some greens like kale are easier to digest when lightly cooked.
- Reach for some raw, organic celery when you crave something crunchy.[71] It's loaded with water and fiber to move toxins out.
- Choose fresh blueberries when you have the option. Blueberries are one of the most nutrient-dense foods and one of the most satisfying. They are loaded with fiber for efficient digestion and they fill you up. If you are trying to slim down, eat a small bowl of blueberries at bedtime to feel satiated until morning.

- Water, Water, Water. Five ways to brighten up your hydration with flavor-enhancing add-in's: a drop of tangerine or other dietary citrus essential oil, sliced cucumbers, fresh fruits like berries or watermelon, peppermint leaves or essential oils for cool energy or traditional wedges of lemon. Add your ingredients to purified water or sparkling if you'd like a little fizz.
- Fruits smoothie vs Veggie smoothie, keep it separate to avoid stress on digestive tract: Fruit smoothie: 1/2 C frozen berries, 1/2 C water, herbal tea or coconut water Veggie smoothie: 1 C greens (spinach, parsley or baby kale), 1/2 avocado, 1/2 cucumber, 1/2 C water or coconut water, few ice cubes added to thicken.
- Add spice: Turmeric is a super spice, found to lower inflammation in many studies. This traditionally Indian spice pairs well with curry sauces, meats and veggies.[72]
- Eat a spoonful of local honey each day to strengthen your immune system. Studies have shown it to have a positive effect on many body systems including plasma.[73] While eating a lot of sugars can stress your body, trading out white sugar for the honey can be a good step toward positive changes.
- Pack up a Superfoods Mix. Combine a handful of each: Almonds, Walnuts, Dried blueberries, wolf berries,[74] sunflower seeds, pumpkin seeds. Store in an airtight container for quick energy when you're busy.
- Drink fresh almond or cashew milk.

Nut milks are easy to make, just soak in water overnight-stir in a blender. Strain through cheesecloth. Refrigerate. *Bringing whole foods into your meal planning gives you a connection with it's source. It gives perspectives into how easy some of it is to make. Once you discover the simplicity of pure ingredients, the choices are easier to make.*

- Replace traditional dairy foods for a day, week or month with an alternative: almond, coconut or rice sources. Dairy foods encourage mucous formation and may slow down your body's natural cleansing function.[75]
- Eat organic soy products in moderation if at all. Soy is a natural source of estrogen that may support female hormones, so men, boys and small children can skip this ingredient.
- Choose natural sweeteners like honey, 100% maple syrup, dates or coconut sap sugar that enhance the flavor of your food or beverage, not just sweetening it. Skip white sugars, corn syrup and other highly processed sugars that are hard on kidneys.[76]
- Eat freshly prepared meat and fish. Use moderation with those that are naturally preserved. Skip deli meats and sausages cured with sulfites which might trigger allergic reactions.[77]
- Make your own salad dressing with fresh ingredients. It's super easy and satisfying.

DIY Salad Dressing is as simple as mixing together:

1 tsp Balsamic vinegar
2 tsp Olive oil

Pinch of Celtic Sea salt
Fresh cracked pepper to taste

- Make your own chicken broth (see recipes in the resource section)
- Shred your own cheese (see what to avoid with shredded cheeses below)

Foods to Exclude or Avoid

- Avoid self-destruction foods: processed, fast food, sugar, alcohol, coffee, soda, breads, pastas and other carbs, & dairy for some people.
- Use sugar in moderation. When you do, appreciate it as an indulgence like in a rich piece of specialty chocolate that you savor.
- Be aware of possible food allergies or sensitivities. The most common mood triggering ingredients are man-made or genetically modified: corn, wheat, soy, artificial colorings, preservatives and flavorings. Aside from being non-nutritive, these ingredients have been linked to a host of allergic symptoms including irritability, inability to focus, and hyperactivity.[78]
- Products labeled with the ingredient "spices" may contain man-made flavorings you'll want to avoid. Most soups, snacks and packaged mixes contain MSG or Monosodium Glutamate. MSG has produced a long list of side effects the years it's been in production (which continues to grow each year in the US as it is found in more and more foods) studied for it's negative effects on the human body and brain including it's propensity to trigger depression.[79]
- Pre-shredded cheddar cheese is usually coated with silicone dioxide or cellulose fibers that keep it from sticking, but may increase your chances of forming a kidney stone.[80] Natamycin is added to pre-shredded cheeses, an antibiotic to prevent mold production. Wait, isn't cheese mold?? Of course it is, and in many countries like France the different molds are revered for their delicacy to the palate and also nourish your gut flora, but feared in the ultra-sanitized diets of Americans. Rightly so, as mass-produced cheeses do bear a higher risk of growing harmful bacteria like listeria. Besides giving you a connection to your food, shredding your own cheese tastes fresher and you'll avoid those silly additives that make it convenient to use.
- Avoid additives like carageenan. this is a seaweed used as a thickener for processed milks. It is also used in research, fed

to lab animals to induce inflammation to test the effectiveness of pharmaceutical drugs against inflammation.[81]

- Non-organic soy is one of the most sprayed crops as a GMO resistant to Round Up weed killer.[82] Julie Ross of the Mood Cure writes that soy is hard to digest and may impair digestion of other critical nutrients. Additional research has shown it's negative impact on thyroid function[83] and hormones including a decrease of testosterone in males who consumed soy[84] as well as impaired brain function and links to Alzheimers.[85] The more tofu consumed, the more impaired the brain.[86] Many traditional salad dressings, pasta sauces and pre-packaged dinner mixes are also made with soybean oil, so make your own to avoid to avoid this source.
- Farmed Atlantic Salmon is more likely to contain antibiotics and growth hormones to increase production.[87]
- Celery is on the Dirty Dozen list of most highly pesticide-sprayed crops.
- Limit yeast and yeast products which might contribute to overgrowth in the body. "Candida" is a common source of urinary tract infections and acne. Consuming yeast products and sugar feed this organism.[88]
- Skip artificial sweeteners like aspartame. These are just sweet flavored chemicals linked with many side effects, and they're just not natural.
- Pass on the artificial spreads and go for the real butter. Some of these spreads have a chemistry similar to plastic, yuk!
- Avoid alcohol. Aside from dulling your pre-frontal cortex, the area that affects our reasoning and decision making skills, alcohol has been linked with numerous diseases including cancer, and because it restricts blood flow to the brain, affects learning, motor skills and abilities to manage stress.[89] Overuse of alcohol has also been linked with

potential decrease in Serotonin,[90] a hormone that keeps your brain happy.

- Read labels and when you reach for the box or can, choose products with ingredients you know. Skip the ones with long chemical names. Most of these are additives that will confuse your chemistry, slow down your metabolism and train your taste buds to crave the processed ingredients.

Each American consumed over 100 pounds of sugar in the year 2012, and the number continues to rise as we trade soda for coffee and sugared yogurts. The average soda carries 39 grams of sugar, the caramel-macchiato coffee drinks may contain 34+ grams of sugar. Some flavored yogurts are now carrying just as much sugar as the soda and specialty coffee drinks so READ THOSE LABELS!

Some Great To-Do's

- Build a Healthy Relationship with Food. Keep a journal to note your intake along with any emotions you're feeling so you can identify when you might be eating emotionally. When you catch yourself heading down this path, re-direct to a non-food activity like going for a walk, gardening or another hands on activity that gets your body moving.
- Make a meal from scratch to be connected to your food from start to finish. You can choose the ingredients and prepare them in a nourishing way that's fresher than any takeout. Cooking your own meal also gives you an appreciation for the process and you'll skip a lot of preservatives and flavorings in the process. (My favorite down to earth, healthy cookbooks: The Moosewood Cookbook by Molly Katzen, Nourishing Traditions by Sally Fallon, and Whole Foods for the Family, Roberta Bishop Johnson.)
- Treat yourself to some healthy sweets instead of trans fat baked goods. Fresh fruit with coconut cream and a pinch

of cinnamon can satisfy your sweet tooth and nourish your body. A piece of dark chocolate is a better choice (and packed with antioxidants) than sugar-filled milk or caramel chocolates. Take notice when you are drawn to emotional eating, have a go-to list of alternative activities to divert you from over-eating in those moments. Keep the list somewhere prominent in your kitchen. Maybe by your chocolate supply :).

- Enjoy slow-food. Cook your foods in the oven or on the stove, even for re-heating. In our instant-society, we expect everything to happen quickly. When we slow down in our day to day routines it gives us space to breathe, reflect and appreciate the normalcy of routines. Daily routines keep us in the present.
- Use antibiotics only when necessary. Many antibiotics will kill good bacteria which may impact your brain cell development as.[91]

Supporting Healthy Digestion

As mentioned earlier, the gut is often called the "second brain" because of it's complex wiring between the nervous system and the brain,[92] functioning at an involuntary level digesting foods, absorbing nutrients, protecting the immune system and eliminating waste. The gut is also referred to as the "seat of the emotions" because of it's effect on simple and complex mental functions. Most of the body's Serotonin, the happy hormone that regulates our mood, is also produced in the gut. Those suffering from depression or anxiety are often low in Serotonin, but it's functions go beyond regulating our mood. It's function has also been linked with blood clotting, bone density, liver regeneration and function of libido.[93] Eating well can not only take care of your gut biome, it can be beneficial to your brain health since 90% of our body's Serotonin is found in our digestive tract. Some depressive disorders have even been treated by stimulating the Vagus Nerve which is inter-connected with the digestive organs[94]. The Vagus Nerve pathways between the brain and organs is what gives us our "gut feelings that signal what is safe, life sustaining, or threatening, even if we cannot quite explain why we feel a particular way." [95] Because of these deep-rooted connections, keeping your emotional health balanced can affect your digestion and likewise, an upset stomach can impact our psyche. Improve your digestion and you'll be more likely to think clearer, manage stress, and feel better overall.

The Vagus Nerve is the second largest nervous system in the body, second to the Central Nervous System in the spinal chord. The Vagus Nerve connects many of the tissues in our main organs, including those in the digestive tract, with the brain stem. There are constant signals coming from the Vagus Nerve to the brain relaying information back and forth that are critical to healthy bodily functions. At the core of our digestive health is obviously our stomach and intestines, but also includes our liver and kidneys which help to stimulate digestive enzymes and filter and eliminate toxins to name a few functions. All of these intricate designs of our body influence the digestions of foods and assimilation of nutrients to support our overall health. At the center of these systems rest a unique ecosystem involving our gut flora or bacteria.

Our gut flora is organized around a very delicate biome in your digestive tract. Scientists have found healthy humans have 10 times more microbial bacteria in their body than human cells in their body.[96] A great deal of those bacteria thrive in our gut. This "gut flora" includes good bacteria that can support your immune system, brain function and influence all other body systems including the Vagus Nerve.[97] This is so important when you are trying to make better choices in health and wellness.

Feed your body good foods and you will support healthy thinking as well.

Just as your gut flora impact your brain function, the thoughts you have can make a positive or negative impact on your gut health.

How you are thinking when you eat is almost as important as what you eat.

Take time to eat in a sense of calm. This makes your digestive organs work at their best. Did you know there are studies that find when we are eating in stressful conditions, it actually affects the digestive juices released to process our food? When we are in fight/flight/freeze mode, our digestion slows.[98] Ongoing stress may even impact the health of our gut, being a major factor in such illnesses as Irritable Bowel Syndrome (IBS), stomach acid imbalances (GERD and Acid-Reflux), ulcers and leaky gut syndrome.[99] The gut-brain connection is very important in preserving your overall health and stress can cause a cascade of imbalances that often lead to these diseases. Those with a damage to or a sluggish Vagal Nerve may show symptoms of digestive distress including gastroparesis, difficulty swallowing or speaking, slow digestion or difficulty managing stress. Yes, there are formal treatments for many of these, but it makes sense to take action where you can to lessen stress in your daily routines and be mindful of the foods you're eating to prevent problems when you are able. Breath patterns for example, can also have a direct positive impact on Vagal function so make sure you take deep, full breaths throughout the day and especially in between bites at the dinner table. It's also important to fully chew your food and take your time. Don't multi-task during meals, watch tv, work on your computer or have intense conversations if you can help it.

Stress + food = stomachache

Undigested foods = malabsorption

These small "stressors" can add up to indigestion over time if they are part of your everyday routines.

Instead, take time to eat your meals in quiet when you can, make your plate pretty, and eat with your eyes. Enjoy the smell, taste and textures of your meal combined with regular breath patterns. Make it a habit to create special components to your mealtimes. It doesn't have to be a fancy five-course meal to be special: use real dinnerware and cloth napkins instead of paper plates, set a placemat under your setting. Place a few flowers in a vase at the center of the table. Turn off the tv and enjoy your meal with a friend or family member. Take this time to build relationship with yourself and others as a space to nourish your body and your soul.

The steps you take to bringing calm emotions to your dinner table are so important to the health of your mind and your body. Our sympathetic nervous system is what revs us up into fight or flight mode. The Parasympathetic Nervous System (PNS) is what calms us down. The Vagal Nerve is the pilot of the PNS so stimulating this nerve keeps it active and alert, ready to soothe your system when the stress passes, allowing our digestive system to operate properly and digest the foods we're eating. Deep breathing is one of the easiest steps you can take to keep your Vagal Nerve and digestive system functioning at their best.

Researchers are collecting mounting information on all the ways our digestive health affects the entire body. We know that the core of our digestive health is obviously our stomach and intestines, but digestion also relies on our liver and kidney health to stimulate digestive enzymes, filter and eliminate toxins to name a few functions. Scientists have even identified a link between some organs and our emotional state. The liver is commonly associated with anger when it is overloaded with toxins. It's not surprising when you understand the physiology of the liver. The liver filters out toxins we are exposed to - chemicals we ingest, breathe in and apply to our skin. The kidneys also filter waste. When your liver and kidneys become saturated with junk they begin to overflow this waste back into your system where it begins to re-circulate. This can create a cascade of unpleasant problems, the least of which will most likely make you feel crummy.

What Are The Side Effects?

A common question doctors ask before prescribing some medications is whether or not you are on medications or have liver or kidney disease. It doesn't matter if it's an acne lotion, anxiety treatment or anti-fungal meds. Over-the-counter and prescription medications often put stress on these organs because they are working to eliminate the chemicals in the drug as soon as you ingest it, breathe it in or apply it to your skin. One of the main tests pharmaceutical manufacturers place on their drugs prior to FDA approval is to gauge the effects on your main detoxing organs, the liver and the kidneys. In developing drugs, manufacturers assess three main affects:

1. What the drug does to the body
2. What the body is doing to the drug
3. ADME **Absorption** into related areas: ingestion, topical, inhalation or intravenous use, **Distribution** of drug into the bloodstream, **Metabolism** of the drug and affect on enzyme production from the liver, and **Elimination** affects on the kidneys.

Have intelligent conversations with your doctor about what medications are really essential for your situation. It can be easy to fall into taking a cascade of prescription drugs that are only dealing with symptoms and not reaching to a root cause. This does call for some patience on our end to consider if we are having a real challenge or just responding to a more temporary stimulus in our surroundings. If you are on prescription medications, it's important to be even more vigilant about chemicals you might be exposed to around your home and in personal care items. Even essential oils and some herbs may stress the liver and kidneys if taken in large quantities or when combined with pharmaceuticals. Treat these natural substances just like you would alcohol or another drug, don't mix them!

There are so many healthy alternatives to non-emergency situations, some have endured the rigors of time, like good old-fashioned chicken soup for soothing your mind and body during simple health challenges like a common cold or recovery after a surgery. (you'll find the recipe in the back section of this book). Find a doctor who is familiar with these simple health-supporting strategies.

Practical Choices To Support Your Digestive Tract

- Drink fresh squeezed lemon juice in a cup of warm water the first thing in the morning to wake up and purify your digestive tract.
- Keep your plumbing clear, don't hold it: use the bathroom when you need to. Holding it keeps your body from removing those toxins from your body when it's needed. Need some natural help? Make sure you have a good calcium-magnesium supplement which relaxes your muscles to let go of waste. Foods that can help naturally include coconut, dates, figs, prunes and apples.
- Go without gluten or grains for a day, week or month and note any changes in your energy, digestion and mental clarity.[100]
- Supplement your diet with natural vegetable oils like olive, coconut, sesame and palm oil. Margarine, shortening and artificial fats are difficult to digest and slow down your metabolism. Good fats boost it. Avoid canola oil which is genetically modified. It was engineered in the 1960's from rapeseed oil seed and often grown as the Round Up Ready variety which would produce an oil with pesticide residue on it.[101] [102]
- Have a picnic anywhere, eat some watermelon. Watermelon has a cleansing effect on the body and carries toxins along with it. Do this on an empty stomach so it moves through more efficiently.[103]
- Drink fresh juices for a day. Let your digestive tract rest for 12-24 hours and just drink fresh made juices like carrot, apple, beet and ginger. Fresh sprouts are loaded with

vitamins and minerals. They also may bind to heavy metals, supporting the liver and kidneys in waste elimination.[104]

- "An apple a day keeps the doctor away." Ben Franklin. Apples contain pectin that binds them to heavy metals and moves them out. Regular apple consumption may also soften gall stones and help them pass smoothly out of your system.

- Crush the garlic, it's gentle on your intestinal flora but powerful against unhealthy microbes. Garlic may also bind to and neutralize some heavy metals. It's also great for heart health.[105 106 107]

- Digestive health = skin & brain health. Cardamom, fennel, ginger, peppermint, turmeric and garlic are all natural soothers to the digestive tract. Add these spices to your entrees, drink them in teas or mix up an essential oil blend and massage gently over the belly.

- Have a simple salad: lots of greens with a squeeze of fresh lemon juice, a drizzle of olive oil and a pinch of sea salt.

- Take a break from meat. Animal proteins put stress on the kidney. You'll give your kidneys a break and your digestive tract will run more efficiently. Trade out the animal proteins for some plant sources: nuts, seeds, legume, and eggs.

- Add fermented foods to your diet. There are thousands of good gut bacteria in our systems, one of the most prevalent are the *Lactobacillus* strains.[108] Lactobacilli naturally occur on cabbage which makes fermented veggies and sauerkraut a good source of these pro-biotics. Yogurts are typically not a significant source of the microbes, especially if you've ever been on antibiotics. There are also some great pro-biotic beverages like Kombucha. Just make sure the probiotics are listed separately in the ingredients. Look for products that contain at least four or more different flora to really get the best benefit from them.

Simple DIY Fermented Veggies
http://bit.ly/FermentedVEGGIES

Whole Foods For Your Liver And Kidneys

- Naturally cleanse your kidneys with foods that have gentle
  diuretic and purifying qualities: celery, cranberries (fresh),
  cucumbers, lemons, parsley, watermelon.[109][110]
- Mid-day pick up: Eat some fresh grapefruit or squeeze the
  fresh juice. Grapefruit is very cleansing to the digestive tract
  and may even boost metabolism. Studies have found that
  drinking fresh grapefruit juice may make you less prone to
  developing kidney stones.[111] Citrus fruits are also mood
  boosters, giving you a slice of sunshine.[112][113] If you are on
  prescription medications, check with your pharmacist to
  make sure the meds don't interact with the grapefruit juice
  which is a common reactor to drugs.
- Save your corn on the cob for the summertime when you
  can find a local organic farmer. Traditionally grown corn is
  a common GMO crop that may stress the kidneys. If you
  have any kidney issues, skip corn and corn products
  altogether. Corn is often used in gluten-free packaged
  goods so read your labels.[114]

**Corn starch is used as a thickener in packaged goods
(think puddings, sauces, soups, prepackaged dinner
mixes), absorption of moisture in grains and spices.
Read your labels so you can avoid those corn fillers and
replace with natural thickeners like chia seeds and
arrowroot powder. Recipe for Chia Seed pudding with
almond milk.**

- Add shredded raw beets to your salad or drink them in a
  fresh juice. Beets support a healthy liver. In juices, they
  combine well with carrots, ginger and lemon.
- Add parsley to everything. It's a natural breath freshener

and supports liver and kidney health. In juices the flavor complements lime. Aside from making the food on your plate look like a Pinterest post, it's packed with important B-vitamins, potassium, magnesium and calcium. The nutrients are at their prime when you eat it fresh.

- Make ginger tea: finely chop 2 teaspoons of fresh ginger and steep a few minutes in hot water. Ginger is a super food! It supports digestion, calms irritation in the intestines and purifies the liver and kidneys. It's packed with important nutrients: potassium, copper, and magnesium. (Caution, do not use ginger if you are currently on the medication Warfarin which could result in severe bleeding).
- Add lemons to your plate whenever you can. Packed with Vitamin C, they purify and support a healthy liver.

Skip Liver-Taxing Substances When You Can

- Heavy metals, pesticide sprayed produce, chemicals in home and person care products, alcoholic beverages, Illicit drugs, over the counter medications and prescription drugs, cosmetics, anti-perspirants, steroids: topical and oral, vaccine adjuvants (additives that stimulate your body's immune response to vaccine ingredients).
- Use natural remedies intelligently to support a healthy body instead of relying on over the counter meds to treat every discomfort you might have. Save the drug use for when you really need it or it's recommended by your doctor. Prescription drugs have a place when there is a health crisis, but ongoing, casual use may tax your liver and kidneys. Have intelligent conversations with your doctor about your options. Be aware of any natural food interactions with any medications you are on, like grapefruit juice which can negate the effects of a drug or peppermint essential oil which may enhance the effects of a drug.
- Replace traditional cosmetics with natural options

- Use an aluminum-free deodorant, avoiding anti-perspirants which block your body's natural response to eliminate toxins through your skin.
- Be informed about vaccines, their ingredients, risks and need for your particular situation. Vaccine ingredients have only been tested for individual components. No vaccines have been researched for their combined effect when 2 or more vaccines are administered at the same time.
- Pay attention to how you feel after eating certain foods. Chocolate, tomatoes, rich meats and sauces may affect liver and gall bladder function. Keep a food journal for a week and avoid any foods you notice sensitivity to.
- Limit or eliminate your intake of large fish like Mahi Mahi and tuna. The larger the fish, the more likely they have accumulated large amounts of heavy metals in their tissues over their long life.
- Avoid soybean and corn oil. Both of these oils are growing in quantity as food additives in many processed foods including salad dressings, pasta sauces, snack foods and condiments, even organics! Soy and corn are some of the most grown GMO (Genetically Modified Organisms) crops. These plants are engineered to withstand the spraying of pesticide residue, known as Round-Up Ready Soy or Corn, leaving pesticide residue on the produce that may stress your detoxifying organs. The active ingredient in the pesticide, glyphosphate, has been found in consumer goods including cereals, baby food and even organic foods.

A Cup of Tea

Temple monks were the first to organize a ceremony surrounding tea drinking in China. It was a simple ritual designed to teach respect for nature, to express humility, and to encourage a sense of peace. Tea is nourishing to the physical body, but the practice can be nurturing to your spirit. Drinking tea spans many cultures where it is often shared with family or friends. It's sometimes taken mid-day during a period of rest and reflection. It can also be used to hydrate the body, bring comfort and extend healing when made with medicinal herbs. From 2007 to 2012, more than 5,600 studies related to tea were produced including studies showing their benefits to many body systems including overall health, weight loss, heart health, the microbiome and your gut health.[115] Make sure you avoid caffeinated teas after 2pm which can disrupt your body's natural sleep cycle. Caffeine content of different teas can vary greatly, even by brand.

Take time to heat the water in a tea kettle rather than popping a cup of water into the microwave. It doesn't take much more time and you'll add an element of delayed gratification that can enhance the ritual of tea time. Choose a tea to suit your mood, focus your thoughts, or keep it simple with black, oolong or green which is packed with antioxidants.[116] For a quick cup of tea, you can use a ready-to-use tea bag. For a more sensory experience, use loose tea and prepare it for steeping on your own, inviting in all your senses.

- Calming teas: chamomile (avoid if you're allergic to ragweed), hibiscus, valerian.
- Energizing: Orange, peppermint, raspberry.
- Cleansing: Burdock, dandelion, milk thistle, red clover Immune supporting: Echinacea, elderberry, ginger, lemon, turmeric.
- Antioxidant rich: Turmeric, licorice, burdock, green, white, rooibos.

Put together a tea tasting. Choose a country and sample teas from different regions in that country: Black teas of India from Niligiri, Assam, and Darjeeling or Ceylon (Sri Lanka) grown in low, middle, and high elevations, Green teas from around the world, Choose the same type of tea, but varying grades of quality.[117]

- Use your 5 senses to bring your tea experience into the

present and help create some positive memories with the smells and flavors of your tea. This simple exercise can help create a sense of calm that you can continue to pair with that cup of tea in the future.

- Look at the dry leaves: what is their color, size and shape? Are they broken or uniform?
- Smell the dry leaf: what aroma is it giving off even before steeping? What memories might be associated with this if at all?
- Touch the tea leaves and notice the texture of their dryness. Do they feel fragile or paper like? or rough and rigid?
- Listen to the water boiling whether you have it in a tea kettle or in an electric pot.
- Savor the taste of the tea and and notice if the flavors change as the tea settles down after steeping. Are you drawn to sweeter teas, lighter or more bold flavors? Write down any observations you make.

Further Reading and Cooking Resources

Good, Clean Food. Lily Kunin

Moosewood Cookbook. Molly Katzen

Nourishing Traditions. Sally Fallon

The Nourished Kitchen. Jennifer McGruther

Prescription for Nutritional Healing. Phyllis A. Balch 11

Fasting

The first time I fasted I was 7 months pregnant. Our pastor encouraged everyone in our church to fast for 10 days and pray. I knew that eliminating food for the next 10 days wouldn't be feasible. I had heard about fasting but never learned about it the way he described. Some could choose a traditional fast which eliminated all food, but we were also encouraged to fast from anything. It wasn't about being legalistic and following a set of rules. What mattered was our heart condition as we followed the fast.

Fad diets starve us for short time periods in order to achieve a slimmer waistline for a deadline. Fasting in faith completely connects your mind, body and spirit as you deny your earthly desires of something and meditate in faith. Fasting can be as simple as denying yourself a daily cup of coffee at that drive-thru place that charges $4 a cup for a 500 calorie indulgence. Save up the money you would spend on take-out coffee for a week or month and donate it to a good cause. Our youth group pastor did this a few times to inspire students to give up something to save for. The students raised over $10,000 and were able to purchase a private well for a village in Bangladesh. That's fasting with a purpose!

One of the goals of fasting can be to observe your heart and mind in the process. It's not what you fast, it's how you do it. Pick anything. When I was pregnant I loved chai tea, indulgent with whole milk and a lot of sugar. It was comforting and I knew it would be good to remove it from my life for a short period. I figured I could make it 10 days, easy. Wrong. I was shocked at how tough it was to hold off on my cravings for that sweetness throughout the day. The following 10 days were an eye opening experience into the many times I desired that cup of tea for comfort instead of reaching out in faith to Jesus. It was a crutch of sorts, not quite as addicting as cigarettes. But fasting, or "taking a break from it" opened my eyes to how I was being led by longings of my physical body without concern of my mind and spirit. How often do we pass through our days making choices with little thought as to why we do them or what is influencing us? Fasting can give us insight into those areas so we can break tradition and move onto more intentional self-care that fosters healthy relationships with God, ourselves and others. If you'd like to have a positive experience with fasting, look at it as a tool to better self-awareness in your mind, physical body and in faith. Yes, fasting is often about removing something physical from our lives, but it disrupts our day to day challenging us to observe our mind and spirit and faith in each moment.

Chapter 11: Be Beautiful

YOU AS THE MASTERPIECE

You are a piece of artwork, created in the image of God. And you were empowered to make the most of that Masterpiece the moment you were born. You can take any trials, difficulties or heartaches and make it into something beautiful. It might be to help someone else in a similar situation, or just to persevere and see your strength. Taking care of your physical body and understanding what keeps you healthy will help you keep your mind strong with clearer thinking so you'll continue to make the best choices you can.

Choosing The Best "Art" Supplies

Not all body care products, essential oils, supplements and foods are the best for everyone. I lovingly encourage you to discover what will be best for you. If you find a positive experience from something specific, repeat and add it to your daily routine. If something doesn't agree with you (possibly from a negative memory from an aroma in a product) don't force it into your life because you feel that you should. Don't be afraid to invest in good things. If you had a Maserati in your driveway, you wouldn't put cheap fuel in it. How much more valuable are you, your mind and your spirit? Invest in yourself the best you can with your budget, and consider it an honor to care for your Creator's Masterpiece.

Sometimes instead of investing in more, actually cutting back on products is the better option. My teenage daughter had suffered from acne for years (she may have gotten this from her mom). We have tried almost every product on the market, natural and otherwise I admit. We stopped short of putting her on antibiotics, which I knew was not an option for our family. We finally discovered that many facial products with any fragrance in them other than pure essential oils caused her to break out in addition to using scrubs of any kind. Her very sensitive skin cannot handle the slightest physical sloughing. These are observations we were able to make by tracking her monthly hormones, diet, water intake, sleep and stress. Just these casual observations helped us to identify the culprits that would send her skin into an inflamed state. You'll be discovering little nuances in your physical, emotional and spiritual perspectives as you explore these tips. I encourage you to journal, observe and adopt what routines align with the fullness of who you are.

Choices to Care for Your Body

- Take a nap. Our perspectives are always better when we are well-rested.
- Ditch the scale and measure your weight by how your clothes fit.
- Remove the mirrors. Mirrors serve a purpose, but too many of them make it tempting to overanalyze our physical selves when we see our reflection everywhere we turn.
- Cover it up. Culture says we will develop confidence if we reveal our body. I challenge you to consider these perspectives and how they fit with your own self-esteem.
- Celebrate your unique qualities, write them down. Keep a file of your accomplishments that are not tied to your physical body.
- Write down a list of 3 character traits you like about yourself. Add one more that you'd like to work on in the

coming weeks. Some ideas: caring, generous, thoughtful, honest, loyal, reliable, trustworthy, brave, reverent, friendly, helpful, positive.
- Take a break from looking at magazines and catalogs that influence our perspectives of what women look like.
- Celebrate your imperfections as unique qualities that make you beautiful.
- Have a sense of humor at times. Taking ourselves too seriously all the time is stressful.

Pamper Your Skin

- Skin care recipes: scrubs. Exfoliate your skin with a Sea Salt Scrub: 1/4C pure Celtic Sea Salt (fine) mixed with 1/4 C organic olive oil, 3-4 drops of essential oils of your choice. Soothing skin oils = Chamomile, Lavender, Geranium, Ylang Ylang, Sandalwood, Myrrh, Helichrysum.
- Stop using skin care and facial products for one week, let your skin breathe. Give your skin a weekend skin renewal (link)
- Give yourself a cleansing facial with French Green Clay, aloe vera and essential oils. Calming essential oils = Chamomile, Frankincense, Lavender. Hydrating Essential Oils = Copaiba, Geranium, Myrrh, Sandalwood.

- Massage skin with finely ground almonds, crushed rose petals and olive oil to soften and smooth rough skin.
- Purifying Facial Mask: Simple DIY with Bentonite Clay Powder or Rhassoul Clay, water or Aloe Vera and 2-3 drops essential oils of your choice. Purifying essential oils = Rosemary, Tea Tree, Cypress.
- Coffee Grounds exfoliation: Massage your body with organic coffee grounds to brighten skin and slough off dead skin cells. Mix 1/4 cup organic coffee grounds with 1/4 cup of organic olive oil. Add 1-2 drops of essential oils and

massage over areas in a circular motion. Rinse with warm water.

- Dry brush your skin to improve circulation and lymph flow. Start at the feet and work up the legs, to the arms and the body always brushing towards the heart. You can dry brush anytime, but doing it in the morning before a shower is a great way to wake up your system for the day.
- Find out what is in your skin-care and beauty products. Ignorance is not bliss if it leads to disrupted hormones or thyroid issues. Check out www.EWG.org/SkinDeep/ to find out how your products rank and to find cleaner options.

Hair

- Hair Brightener: Wash hair with 1 Tablespoon of baking soda mixed in a cup of warm water. This will not suds! Massage through the scalp to remove product build up and toxins from shampoo and styling products.
- Rinse Hair and remove soap residue with a refining hair rinse: mix 1 tsp apple cider vinegar in 1/2 gallon of warm water and pour over hair for a final rinse.
- Switch your liquid body soap with a natural bar soap. Most liquid soaps (except for natural Castile soap) have harsh chemicals to fragrance, color, thicken and preserve the liquid.

Relaxation

- Take an Epsom Salt or Magnesium Salt Bath. Ancient Minerals is my favorite brand, add 2 Cups salts and 5 drops food grade, therapeutic lavender essential oil to a warm bath. Soak for at least 30 minutes, rinse quickly in a cool shower. Wrap up immediately in a robe or cotton clothing and immediately lie down to rest for at least 1 hour to get the most relaxation benefits from your soak.

- Give yourself a simple leg massage, flowing towards the heart to stimulate your lymphatic system and improve circulation. Essential oils that support healthy circulation = Cypress, Juniper, Marjoram.
- A cleansing kelp bath nourishes your skin. Mix 2-3 Tablespoons organic kelp powder into 1/4 cup warm water. Stir this into a hot bath and soak for 20-30 minutes. Rinse thoroughly with warm water.
- Soak in a tub of sea salt. Mix 1 C natural sea salt (avoid iodized sea salt which is over- processed and void of nutrients and minerals), 1/4 cup baking soda and 3-4 drops of essential oils of your choice.
- Sit in a sauna until you begin to sweat. Make sure to drink plenty of water to replace the lost fluid from sweating.
- Use natural candles that are fragrance-free like beeswax and soy. Candles are scented with chemicals that may trigger asthma and allergies, not what you want for relaxation! These same chemicals have been found in the cord blood of babies so they are like a form of second-hand smoke. Trade out chemical plug-ins and aerosol sprays for a simple essential oil freshener you can make in 2 minutes.

http://bit.ly/airFreshener

- Diffuse natural essential oils to relax and promote a sense of calm in your space. Citrus essential oils are uplifting and purifying, tree oils like cedarwood, sandalwood and frankincense are calming.
- Practice deep breathing techniques with affirming thoughts or prayers to calm your mind. Even regulating your breath as you listen to a piece of calming music can be powerful.

Personal Routines

- Wear natural fibers that breathe like your skin: cotton,

linen, silk, hemp, wool.

- Choose organic clothing when you're able. The cotton industry uses about 16% of the world's supply of pesticides and herbicides.[118] Cotton is one of the most sprayed crops with pesticides and each time we have opportunity to support organic it will make the world a better place. Organic clothing is also softer than conventional.
- Refresh your spirit and build in daily time for meditation and prayer. Keep it simple if you need to and just focus on one scripture or verse a day or week. If you need some prompts, pick up a devotional book or start with some of the verses in the back of this book.

Books for Mind, Body, Spirit

Skin & Body Care

Aromatherapy, Valerie Ann Worwood

Uplifting stories, quotes and musings

One Thousand Gifts, Ann Voskamp

Positive Thinking

Battlefield of the Mind. Joyce Meyer

Discipline and the Glad Surrender. Elisabeth Elliot

Intentional Living, John Maxwell

The Journey of Desire. John Elderidge

Soul Keeping. John Ortberg

Chapter 12: Be Nurturing

CREATING A PURE HOME AND BODY

Essential Oil Care

Creating nurturing routines for yourself is one way to stay faithful in your pursuit of health, strength and peace. You don't have to spend a lot, just invest in some simple tools and bring on the love. For the cost of a spa facial or treatment, you can invest in a great starter set of essential oils that will keep on giving for weeks after your purchase. Give yourself a little bit of care every day when you have quality beauty resources on hand. By trading out synthetic fragrances in personal care products for those containing pure essential oils, you'll have a safe and holistic experience.

Pure oils come from plant material which our bodies readily absorb. They are highly valued because it takes many pounds of plant material to produce just a small bottle of essential oil. These plant oils are very concentrated and you only need a drop or two for pure aromatic bliss without chemicals. Pure essential oils will not break down over time if they are stored in a cool, dry location. Pure oils should last almost forever if they are stored properly. Aromatherapists will even store rare oils in the refrigerator to preserve them from any possible damage by air or sunlight. Buyer beware, though as there are no regulation keeping a manufacturer from putting synthetic fillers into real plant oils and still calling them "pure" or "therapeutic". Chemical fillers in an essential oil will cause the product to break down over time, if you see an expiration date on an oil bottle, this could be a red flag that there are synthetics in the essential oil. The manufacturer may be encouraging you to use up the product before any breakdown is detected.

Make sure you purchase quality oils from a company you trust. I get my oils from a company that grows their own plants on farms they own and they even distill the plant material on their farms! The company I've worked with has been producing the world's top quality essential oils for over 25 years, setting the standard in chemistry of pure oils from plants grown in ideal conditions and processed properly through distillation. If you'd like to get your oils from this company, check them out! http://bit.ly/wholesaleOILS

When you are using a pure, therapeutic essential oil, your bodies know how to absorb nutrients and antioxidants from these plant oils that work in harmony with the body's chemistry. The positive effects of essential oils on blood circulation are well known. They play an important part in bringing oxygen and nutrients to the tissues while assisting in the efficient disposal of waste products that are produced by cell metabolism.[119] Essential oils make great natural resources for the simplest, purest skin and body care that no man-made chemicals can match. They are good for you, and like whole foods for body care. When you choose to treat your body as a temple, consider all the possibilities for trading out man-made chemicals for these beautiful plant extracts that will nourish your senses.

For Specific Spa Recipes, visit the Resources section at the back of the guide

'Essential' Tips

• Massage lemon essential oil into the soles of your feet, seal

192

in with a lavender lotion and cover with cotton socks at bedtime to soften callouses and dry, cracked heels.

- Drink 1 drop of food grade, lemon essential oil in a glass of water when you travel to keep your immune system strong. Make sure your essential oil is labeled as a Dietary Supplement.

- Skip the scented body lotions and massage your body with organic sesame oil BEFORE a shower or bath. Use soap sparingly to keep the skin hydrated. Sesame oil massage is an Ayurvedic practice that nourishes the body and mind in full relaxation. Sesame oil helps to tame inflammation in the body and hydrates over dry skin.

- Massage grapefruit or lemon essential oil into areas of cellulite to improve skin appearance. Make sure you avoid sun exposure after, though. Citrus essential oils increase your sensitivity to the sun and potential to burn. Mix 2 drops of grapefruit essential oil with 1 teaspoon vegetable carrier oil like sesame, jojoba or apricot oil.

- Rub your feet by applying gentle pressure to the soles of your feet to stimulate reflexology points that affect your whole body. Even better, have someone else rub your feet! Add some soothing essential oils like lavender, chamomile or a blend like YL Stress Away, Dream Catcher or Valor.

- Spritz your toes with *Melaleauca alternifolia*, also known as "Tea Tree oil". This species of plant oil has powerful purifying qualities and can keep the skin on your feet clean and fresh. This is an important step to take if you're using public showers or receiving a pedicure from a spa.

- Make your own foaming soap. The magic is in the foaming pump and all you need is castille soap (My favorite is Dr. Bronner's baby mild, unscented), essential oils and water. Make sure you dilute the soap as it's super concentrated, 1/4 soap to 3/4 water and 10-12 drops of essential oils of your choice. Citrus oils are purifying and make great combinations no matter how you combine them.

http://bit.ly/DIYfoamingSOAP

- Save hand sanitizers for when you have no access to running water. The CDC recommends simple hand washing with soap and water as the most effective way to keep hands clean.[120]

Many essential oils are naturally cleansing, cinnamon, clove, thyme, tea tree and lavender are some of the most powerful purifiers. DIY hand cleaner: mix together 2 ounces aloe vera with 10 drops essential oils of your choice. Add 1-2 drops of a citrus oil to the mix to brighten up aromas and add to the synergy. Fun combinations: Lavender + Peppermint, Cinnamon + Grapefruit, Rosemary + Tea Tree, Lemon + Thyme.
http://bit.ly/DIYhandCLEANER

- Clean without chemicals. Cinnamon, clove, rosemary, tea tree (also known as melaleuca alternifolia) are purifying oils. Mix up your own cleaning spray to wipe down bathrooms, kitchens and work spaces without bleach or chemical cleaners. Dilute equal parts of vinegar and water in a bucket or spray bottle. Add 10-15 drops of essential oils of your choice to the mixture. Spray surfaces and wipe with a clean cloth. Let areas air dry.
- Support your immune system when you trade out man-made chemicals for essential oils. Most essential oils help you relax. When your stress levels are lower, your immune system will be stronger. Just breathing in the purity of essential oils will give you a boost to your psyche as well as your cells.
- Diffuse citrus oils to lift your mood. Lemon, orange and bergamot are some essential oils that have been tested for their abilities to support healthy immune function and alleviate depression.[121]
- Oil Pulling is a traditional Ayurvedic practice to cleanse the

mouth and freshen the breath. It's traditionally used with fennel or peppermint essential oils. After brushing teeth, mix 1 drop of essential oil with a teaspoon of a carrier oil like coconut or sesame oil. Swish mouth for a few minutes, spitting out excess when finished.

- End the day with some calm: copaiba, frankincense and lavender are calming oils that can ease us into a restful night. Apply a drop to your pillow or diffuse a combination that you like to bring on the zzz's.

http://bit.ly/sleepOILS

- Perfume your body with natural plant oils. Their aroma is exquisite and works in harmony with our chemistry. Their support of health and wellness goes beyond the fragrance unlike man-made chemicals. Ylang ylang, jasmine, geranium, chamomile, lavender, sandalwood and spruce all make beautiful aromas that can easily stand on their own as natural fragrance or be combined in a blend for more complex perfume. I like Young Living oils because they have some amazing blends that have been crafted with care and intention.

- Make your own Body Spray. Traditional perfumes are just a combination of synthetic chemicals that are confusing our chemistry. Synthetic perfumes and colognes have been linked with reproductive disorders, endocrine disruption and more. When you create a DIY body spray, you can avoid exposure to these crazy chemicals that may even affect your mood and concentration. Simply fill a 4 ounce glass spray bottle with aloe vera, witch hazel or even purified water with 10-12 drops essential oils of your choice. Spritz on your skin after showering for au natural fragrance.

http://bit.ly/DIYbodySPRAY

- Mix up your own Lotion. Lotions contain many ingredients to emulsify ingredients, preserve the contents or increase absorption. You can mix up a simple moisturizer with just a few ingredients.

http://bit.ly/diyLOTION

- DIY Simple Lip Balm. Moisturize your lips with pure, natural goodness. The easiest recipe you can make is to simply melt a tablespoon of coconut oil, add a drop of lavender essential oil and pour into a glass lip balm container. For a more moisturizing recipe that uses a double boiler.

http://bit.ly/glowingSKIN

- Make your own Tooth Polish. Traditional toothpastes have a lot of fillers and added chemicals to make them foamy and sudsy. When you make your own tooth polish with baking soda, vegetable glycerin, sea salt and natural essential oils you can clean your teeth without all those harsh ingredients.

http://bit.ly/toothPOLISH

"Fruit trees of all kinds will grow on both banks of the river. Their leaves will not wither, nor will their fruit fail. Every month they will bear fruit, because the water from the sanctuary flows to them. Their fruit will serve for food and their leaves for healing." Ezekiel 47:12

Daily Routines in a Green Home

Creating a "green" or natural home is more than a trend to simplify your surroundings. There are definite benefits to our physical bodies and the clearness of our thoughts when we lessen the number of chemicals we are exposed to. Our day to day habits will have a great impact on the energy we have during the day and how well we sleep at night. While it's often easy to disrupt our natural cycles of sleep and wakefulness, it can take much longer to restore them to healthy patterns. But are we making this more complicated than it needs to be? Jean Valnet, MD, a pioneer of Aromatherapy states it simply that "natural sleep remains the real treatment for a state of fatigue brought about by staying awake too long."[122] How often are we pushing our bodies beyond their physical capabilities to go without proper rest and expect them to perform at an optimum? I have learned that writing a book goes a long way to disrupting a good night's sleep! :) Seriously, though, our bodies may keep up for a while, especially if we are adding synthetic or natural stimulants, but eventually our body will rebel. Persistent disruption of this system has ill health effects, affecting memory and learning.[123]

Sleep is the time our body eliminates toxins, renews cells and stores up energy for the day and the more natural you can keep it the better all your body functions will operate. Everyone feels better after a good night's sleep. Why is it so difficult to sleep sometimes? Emotional stress, hormones, nutritional deficiencies and physical ailments can all affect our sleep patterns. Sleep aids are one of the top selling over-the-counter meds, but there are many steps you can take to lessen your need for the chemical bandaids. Obviously, there are often situations where sleep aides are helpful if used for a short term. Sleep aides are like antibiotics, overuse of them will only enable your body to become complacent and rely on outside stimulus for survival. Try to avoid using sleep aids which disrupt your body's natural rhythms. Honor you body's natural ebb and flow in rhythms and it will return favor to you in better rest at night and natural energy when you need it.

Nurturing Routines

- Need energy in the afternoon? Try a natural energizer like breathing in peppermint essential oil, going for a walk, or drinking citrus water.

- Avoid caffeinated beverages after 2pm which can interrupt sleep patterns.
- Take a nap if your schedule allows. Rest when your body calls for it. If you lose sleep a night or two, your body's clock builds in some grace to make up the lost sleep within the next seven days.
- Wear organic cotton pj's and avoid fire retardant finishes.
- Sleep on an organic mattress with natural or organic bedding. Fewer chemicals mean less disruptions in your body's chemistry.
- Go to bed at the same time each night if you can. Our body's natural melatonin levels begin to rise around 10pm. If you stay up after this, the adrenals kick in and override your body's clock to go to sleep, you'll get a second wind and may have trouble falling asleep later.
- Traveling over multiple time zones? Carry a spray bottle of melatonin vs pills or capsules. It will absorb quicker into your system. As soon as you board the plane, set your wake and sleep cycle to your destination's time zone. A spritz of melatonin and some essential oils can help lull you into a sleep when it's time.
- Shut down electronics at least 1 hour before bed to try and shift your body out of technology mode into a natural sleep zone. Turn your wi-fi off at night.
- Drink a glass of warm almond milk, herbal or turmeric tea late in the evening to begin to prepare your body for a restful sleep.
- Drink caffeine-free teas or beverages after 2pm. Caffeine consumed after that time may make it more difficult to fall asleep at bedtime.
- Take a warm bath or do some gentle stretching just before bed to unwind and release any stored up energy from the day.
- Diffuse calming essential oils like sandalwood, frankincense, lavender, cedarwood, copaiba, chamomile or vetiver to bring on the zzz's for rest and relaxation. Choose a scent

you like! There are many choices for calming oils, make it a single or blend that suits your personality. Just make sure it's a pure, therapeutic oil with no fillers or synthetics which could interrupt your sleep.[124]

- Vitamins that support a healthy nervous system and protect your body's ability to move into rest mode include B-vitamins, Magnesium, and Vitamin D. Also see foods that support brain health. If your neurons are firing sporadically, it may affect your sleep patterns. (See Resources in the back section)

- Keep your liver healthy (see foods section). A liver that is full of toxins will spill over into the rest of your system and can affect your rest and wake cycles. It's not uncommon for someone with a sluggish liver to wake between 3 and 4 am when the liver may naturally be regenerating.

- Eat lighter foods later in the day. A rich meal late in the evening stirs up energy towards digestion working against your body's natural rhythm to calm down your body before bed.

- When you get a massage schedule it later in the day. Make sure you clear your schedule afterwards so you can prolong the benefits until you climb into bed.

- Reach for natural sleep aids if you need something to settle down: melatonin spray, herbal teas or homeopathic remedies may be worth a try. Coffee cruda is a Homeopathic remedy that may be helpful for someone who has nervous energy and excitement that is interfering with sleep, such as the night before a big event or trip.[125]

- Drink a cup of chamomile, passion flower or valerian tea later in the evening to bring on the calm.

- Essential oils that support sleep: Roman chamomile, Copaiba, Frankincense, Neroli, Rose, Sandalwood, Vetiver, Valerian. In one study, Neroli had a powerful effect on sleep compared to Xanax, a benzodiazepine.[126] Diffuse at bedtime to relax, apply a drop to your pillow or a cotton ball and place near your pillow when you lay down to rest.

http://bit.ly/sleepOILS

Digital Detox

We live in a digital society. We are surrounded with more technology than any other generation in history. Preliminary assumptions are that the long term effects are not significant, but growing research is showing otherwise. ADD and ADHD are so common in children as well as autism and other brain disorders. Anti-depressants are some of the most prescribed medications along with mood balancing drugs. We cannot deny that all these extra electronic waves are affecting our body's natural rhythms and electrical patterns. Our central nervous system is our body's hard-wiring and if there is any interference, physically along the spine or electrically through our brain waves, heart rhythms or even at the cellular level, there will be an impact on our health. Because of these growing influences on the dynamics of our body's core systems it's important to be vigilant in your electronics usage, take time to step away from the cell phone and wi-fi whenever can will not only help you think more clearly, you will be giving your body rest from the bombardment of elec-trical stimulation.

I made a rare visit to a spa the other day and planned to sit in the sauna for half an hour. The spa was beautiful, reclaimed wood, Restoration Hardware style interior with a cushy chair and fluffy carpet in my own private spa room to relax. This was luxury! I was in need of a small break in the week and I knew that 30 minutes would be just the renewal I needed. I could step back from my busy schedule and just breathe in the warmth and aroma of those fresh cedar boards infused into dry, hot air warming my body. The atten-dant explained all the controls and functions of the room, and then informed me I could use my cell phone in the sauna. Just being given permission to use my device put a brief damper on my plans for a secluded thirty minutes of heat-filled bliss and relaxation I had anticipated all week. I actually grabbed my phone (Maybe because I had been given permission to do so at no endangerment to my device) sent one email and realized this would totally defeat the purpose of my visit so I quickly put it back into my backpack. By the time I decompressed from the little scuttle of all this, I was half way through my session. Quick, 17 minutes left, I need to relax, now!

Not.

My week of anticipation for this mind and body-calming appointment evaporated within minutes of taking the option to hold on to my device. The effects couldn't be reversed and the time I had carved out for pampering was cut short. That visit reminded me to embrace every moment I can to fully step away from tech whenever I can for chunks of time. No, five or ten minutes while you go to the bathroom doesn't count. I know that when the phone makes it with me to the bathroom even just to hit "send", it's time to take a break.

When we're not actually using it, our technology creeps into our schedules through our thoughts: do I have it with me? Is it charged? If I'm going out, how and where will I charge it? How much more has the screen cracked since the last use? Is the screen protector peeling? Am I running out of storage? Is your blood pressure rising? Stress. Aside from occupying many of our waking thoughts, all the technology we are surrounded with is confusing our nervous systems and brain function. Yes, the busy-ness of electronic meetings, online shopping and social events can create a hectic schedule, but scientifically, the electronics are interfering with our normal body functioning, causing some things to go haywire in our vision and brain function, so to say.

Socially, the use of electronic devices robs us of intimacy and personal interaction if we rely on it as our primary method of communication. Text messages, emails and IM's do not convey feelings and non-verbal elements of communication that are so important in understanding each other. Overuse of technology devices dulls our skills in social interaction, our abilities to cope with stress and our emotional intelligence. Simply having a cell phone nearby-without even checking it-can reduce empathy.[127] Digital media encourages multi-tasking which leads to "fragmented" thinking.

Researchers at the University of London dramatize how damaging multitasking can be. One study found that participants who multi-tasked during cognitive tasks experienced IQ score declines that were similar to what researchers would expect to see if the study subjects had smoked marijuana or stayed up all night. IQ drops of 15 points for multitasking adults lowered their scores to the average range of an eight-year old child.[128] Not only is multitasking affecting our IQ, the quick communication styles of social media encourage disconnected thinking. Dr. Elias Aboujaoude, director of Stanford University's Impulse Control Disorders Clinic states "The more we become used to just sound bites and tweets, the less patient we will be with more complex, more meaningful information. And I do think we might lose the ability to analyze things with any depth and nuance. Like any skill, if you don't use it, you lose it."[129]

In addition to the behavioral affects that technology use brings on, electronic devices give off an Electromagnetic Frequency, that's EMF for short. All of our body have an electrical impact on the wiring of our our Central Nervous System which impact every body function we have including thought formation and attention, memory, appetite and digestion, hormone function, metabolism, fight and flight responses to name a few. All of our body systems and brain run on electrical signals. Many EMF's interfere with our body's natural electrical patterns which may result in psychological and physiological challenges. These changes are becoming so signifi-cant that some doctors are recommending that schools for younger children limit wi-fi services to small amounts of time in a school day to protect growing and developing brains.[130] Electrical stimulation from cell phone use can even be detected in elevated stress hormones in our saliva[131] and antioxidant levels in the eyes.[132] Numerous studies have been replicated to demonstrate the negative impact that EMF's have on other body systems including decreased melatonin production[133], impact on the blood-brain barrier[134] and eye and ear health[135] to name a few.

The more you can be in natural surroundings and take a break from electronics, the clearer you'll think. Stepping away from the digital as much as you can will keep your nerves calmer and all your body systems will operate as best as they can. While it's helpful to turn off the power every once in a while, it's ideal to do it for larger periods of time so your biological clocks can reset. This is pretty easy if you take a day hike without your phone, go on a vacation for a week or turn off the gear while you sleep and rack up seven to nine hours of down time for your body's natural systems to re-charge. Here are some practical ways to unplug:

- Turn off the Wi-fi at bedtime.
- Leave your device at home for short trips throughout your week.
- Turn off notifications on your phone so you're not tempted to continually check for updates or incoming messages and posts. "Airplane Mode" is best so your device doesn't even vibrate.
- Use speakerphone on your cell to add distance between you and your device. Limit your use of cell phones overall and meet up face to face. This genuine communication really builds healthy relationships and it's good to be with someone! Aside from the human connection you get from a face to face meet up, cell phone use has been shown to disrupt brain wave function resulting in unpredictable brain patterns.[136]
- Charge your phones outside of your bedroom.
- Put space between you and your computer monitor or television screen.
- Follow the 20-20-20 rule when working on the computer to protect your eyesight from longterm damage: Every 20 minutes, focus on an object 20 feet away for 20 seconds.[137]
- Keep your computer monitor 20-30 inches away from your eyes.
- Load an app to your devices to cut down on the glare and promote synchronization with natural lighting. Research has found that prolonged device use during the day increases rate of insomnia. Apps can cut down on the

unnatural blue light of electronics that keep you stimulated.[138]

- Consider getting computer glasses to lessen eye strain

  http://www.allaboutvision.com/cvs/computer_glasses.htm

- Avoid using devices at least one hour before bedtime. Studies show the bright lights and stimulation to your nervous system interfere with melatonin, your body's natural sleep-inducing hormone.[139]
- Supplementing with Vitamin C has shown some potential for protection of the eyes and brain from oxidative stress from electronics exposure.[140]
- When you splurge and get that massage or spa service, leave the electronics behind for the hour and fully immerse your senses in the experience to get the most renewal. If you are able, extend that time to hours or the rest of the day after your treatment to extend the benefits.
- Run through the grass barefoot, take a walk on the beach or a swim in the ocean. The earth is full of positive electromagnetic energy that can actually assist our biological functions in running properly. These beneficial waves can help offset the confusion of the man-made waves not unlike eating whole foods nourishes our bodies unlike processed foods that confuse it. That's why we feel so great on vacations that involve nature.[141] This is referred to by holistic practitioners as "grounding" or "earthing".
- Read an actual book. Not one on your electronic device. Go to a bookstore or library and pick one out. Read it all. If it's your own, add notes, highlight it or mark areas of interest. See how long you can read and keep your attention. Just like exercise, work to extend the time you can focus on the reading of a print book to improve your concentration. Reading a book with characters or biographies of others who have overcome difficulties brings us into better understanding of humanness. We

discover new situations and insights as the characters solve problems and do life in a way that might be different from our own.

"The right book matched with the right person can be the gateway to opening her heart to humanity, to expand the capacity to imagine another's feelings and needs."[142]
-Michele Borba

HOME CARE

- Buy a plant that purifies your air. NASA's top cleaners? Gerbera daisy, Dracaena "Janet Craig", Peace Lily, Bamboo palm and Chrysanthemums.[143]
- Simplify, eliminate clutter and donate unused items in your home. Excess stuff not only creates extra dust, it's visually a distraction. Start small and just clean out a drawer, corner or closet to care for your personal space. Add some fun baskets or organizers to make it visually appealing.
- Replace bleach and harsh cleaning products with natural cleaning products like baking soda, vinegar and essential oils. Just make sure you use essential oils that have no fillers or additives. Smell does not make the oil powerful, it's the chemistry of the undiluted plant oils that carry the power. Scented products and harsh cleaners are just a combination of chemicals that are contaminating our ecosystem.[144] The cleaning potential of pure, plant extracts is unmatched and they have a low impact on our environment and water supplies. A similar comparison would be eating a fresh apple instead of an apple flavored fruit roll up. One is packed with nutrients and antioxidants, the other is just flavor.

Essential oils of clove, cinnamon, thyme and tea tree are

some of the most powerful substances tested against microbes like E.coli and Salmonella.[145]

- Leave your shoes at the door. Removing your shoes at the door is a sign of respect in many cultures. In temples and other sacred spaces, shoes are removed to show reverence. Taking your shoes off when you enter your own home or someone else can show care and attention to the living space. You'll also keep outside dirt and contaminants out of your personal space as your shoes are active petri dishes, collecting specimens everywhere you go.[146]
- Bring in the fresh air: open your windows if you live in a low-pollution area. Off-gassing is the biggest source of indoor air pollution. This happens when chemical from building materials and the stuff we own releases into the air. One of the biggest contributors? Flame retardant finishes & carpets. Open the windows when you can, vacuum carpets regularly and change your furnace air filter at least seasonally.[147]

A Calming Environment

Some days I've got it all pulled together, everything in my schedule runs like clockwork. My expectations fall into place with what was scheduled. Then it can fall apart in a matter of minutes. We've all experienced it, right? That moment when one shift changed everything. No one's struggles are the same, but everyone experiences difficult situations in one way or another. Whether it's a serious family crisis or something lighter and fleeting, our perspectives in the moment can make all the difference in how we hold it together with grace or fall apart.

It was Friday and supposed to be a free day, then gradually my responsibilities filled in until the few moments I might have had evaporated into a Google calendar of red. There was no space in between appointments and obligations. This was going to be uncomfortable. I've been time-challenged my whole life. My creative spirit allows little room for rigidity and scheduling falls into that category. A full calendar has the capability to roll me into a stress ball. Because of this I've learned the hard way to try and build more margin into my life. I'm not happy when those margins are removed, especially if it's not by my choice. This particular Friday our family was running 4 cars for 5 people, 3 with full-time jobs plus two with very flexible changing schedules. A flat tire happens and everything falls apart. My open, free day just got much more complicated. Compromise, unmet expectations, and unknowns could have made my attitude challenged. I admit, I expected to be crabby. Instead, I pushed ahead doing what needed to be done, determined not to let negative feelings creep in or fall apart with an internal temper tantrum over the things I couldn't control. Between stimulus and response is CHOICE.

When your schedule is maxed out and you need better perspective to see the glass "half full", here are some things you can do to stay centered on the tasks at hand, grounded in the present and accomplish what really needs to get done. These tips can help you find rest in the busy-ness without sacrificing your psyche or efficiency.

- **Breathe.** It might seem cliche, but it really works. Breathing not only brings you into the present moment, it fuels oxygen to your brain so you really can think better on your feet when the pressures amount. Exhaling greater than your inhale is a calming breath and super important in those situations where you feel out of control. You can control your breath. If you remember anything, exhale. This is the point your body lets go of what is not necessary at that particular moment.

Focus on some positive words while you do this,
Inhale Love, Exhale, Grace
Inhale Simplify, Exhale Accept

- **Feed your brain good food.** Nutrition is the fuel that can make or break our ability to manage high stress situations. If you're filling up on highly processed foods you'll deprive your brain and body of the energy and nutrients it needs to move through flight mode, making you more likely to crash. Stress reducing foods can assist your body in moving into rest mode after the anxious moments passed. If you have a crazy, busy day ahead, make sure you have a back-up stock of nutrient packed foods high in B-vitamins to keep the calm from the inside out: Sunflower seeds, almonds, walnuts, dried wolfberries, avocados, eggs, lentils and beans.

Super B Calming snack mix
Pick 4 or 5 and mix together: 1/4 Cup each
almonds, Brazil nuts, walnuts, dried wolfberries, dried cherries, currants, dried date pieces, sunflower seeds, pumpkin seeds, dark chocolate chips
Store in airtight container and bring a small amount with you when you're out on the road or traveling.

- **Rest for 10 minutes:** Move into Child's Pose or seated with arms folded on your desk, rest your forehead on your arms. Contact on the forehead calms your central nervous system. Focus on your breath and body during this time, not on your to do list. Make sure you have your phone turned off. We all know that even vibrating phones can be heard, right? Create and honor the quiet, even for a few minutes. (see Child's Pose)
- **Pare away the schedule where you can.** This is the time to look at what is necessary versus what might be frivolous. Trim away so you might gain some margin in the day. Margins give us time to transition from one activity to the next. The more margin you have in between, the more manageable your time will be.
- **Ask for help if it's possible**. This is the time to put

pride aside. No accomplishment is worth self-sacrifice that results in a mental meltdown. You probably have some caring people in your life who are willing to step in to help if you just ask.

- **Stay grounded.** Take a break from technology that isn't essential for the time being. You'll stay focused and have fewer distractions so you can be in the zone for what needs to get accomplished. Being in the zone will help you be most efficient in everything you're doing. Staying grounded can be as simple as being in the present moment in the task at hand. No multi-tasking, checking email or giving social media updates. Put it aside and stay in the game.
- **Say "No".** Where can you simplify your schedule or say no to extra activities? Saying no can help build that sense of calm in your schedule when you (and your family) may need it most.

"Everybody today seems to be in such a terrible rush, anxious for greater development and greater riches. Children have very little time for their parents and parents have very little time for their children and for each other. So the breakdown of peace in the world begins at home"[148]
-Mother Teresa

- **Live locally:** Most communities are filled with social opportunities and dining possibilities. Explore events, businesses and natural resources in your local area for the next few weekends or when the time allows you to explore the spaces nearby. You'll save time driving and give yourself the chances to enjoy the resources close to you.
- **Look for opportunities each day to re-frame your thoughts** and challenge yourself to think outside the box:

Imagine you're in line at the bank, grocery store, doctor. Instead of focusing on the time you are waiting and constantly checking your phone for the time, building frustration with every minute that passes, take the time to text or email someone you care about. Tell them something you are thankful for. If you don't have your phone, write it on a piece of paper. Reframe from entitlement (this line should move faster for the customers - ME) to gratitude (I choose to be thankful for YOU). It doesn't have to be long or complicated, a simple note saying "I am thinking about YOU" can instantly re-frame your thoughts in this moment.

Living With Substance

If only we could see the long term affects of our choices in life as clearly as a price tag on an item at the store, it might make those decisions easier.[149] Yes, there are some seasons in our life when we might rely more on the disposable and convenient items. We did one summer when we moved into a new home. That was a paper plate season. I knew once we were settled into a new routine we'd return to our normal use of the regular plates and we would feel like we were really home. Washing dishes, stacking them in the rack to dry and storing them neatly together on the same shelf seems to form a sense of permanency in our lives. If you are in a paper-plate kind of season, extend yourself grace in this chapter, where you can still dream of the potential to live with fewer disposables.

Innovations and industries have made it instantly economical and easy to toss things in the trash without further thought. Someone else picks up the garbage and transports it to sight unseen where we don't have to deal with it any more. Each time I've been to India I was struck with the reality that many of the people in the most populated country of the world have no formal waste management. They are surrounded by garbage, especially plastic. Residents collect it, sort it and sell it as a precious form of income. I still recall seeing one man riding a bicycle with bare feet. On the back of his bicycle he fastened down a six-foot mound of plastic refuse. He seemed to defy all laws of gravity as he peddled the cargo through the dusty, litter-lined streets. Albeit a bit late, the country put a ban on plastic bags a couple of years ago, but there is still plenty of remaining material to provide ongoing work for tens of thousands of individuals. I think of India almost every time I throw something away. Our oceans have a vortex of plastic garbage that environmentalists are working to eliminate. Plastic waste is a global issue. We all have an impact on this issue. How can we live with less plastic? How quickly do we throw things away out of convenience? In the disposable culture we live in, have we made it quick and easy to throw away other things like friendships, marriages, business relationships? I want to live a life that is filled with substance, relationships worth fighting for, and communities that thrive out of love for each member because each person is valued. So many things are considered disposable and it is time to redeem them!

We are surrounded with plastic. Not only can we find it in almost every consumer goods or packaging, the tiny molecules are entering our water supply from the fibers of our polyester clothing, pharmaceuticals we eliminate in the bathroom, and many other areas too numerous to list here. Because the nature of plastics is confusing our chemistry,[150] any steps we can take to replace it for natural alternatives is helpful. Living with less plastic will take some effort, but it's worth it. You'll gain a deeper appreciation for items of substance. The less we throw away, the more value we place on the things we have: even relationships.

From a scientific perspective, plastics are treated chemicals, many of which have been found to have a negative effect on the body, our water supply, and our environment. In the beginning, God made the plants, the trees, the dirt and man. He did not make poly butyl acrylate. If you're working to create calm in your life it makes sense to remove as many of these chemicals as possible. There is a line, though. No need to become a fanatic. Make the switch to greener pastures a gentle one, a discovery of simpler surroundings made with substance that comes from the Earth: wood, glass, natural fibers.

Life-Honoring Elements

Love can be shattered like glass, but it is beautiful when cared for, polished, protected. But glass is not always convenient. We've had young children in our home for many years and our children have learned to handle glass. Glass breaks. It always seems to happen at the most inconvenient time. Those five minutes before we're rushing out the door, the glass gets knocked off the counter by a passing elbow. A careless move, a distraction and CRASH! Shards of glass everywhere. Some glass breaks in safety size pieces, others explode into thousands of bits and shards. I like to go barefoot in our home when the weather is warm and inevitably the soles of my feet find the one remaining microscopic shard on the well-worn wood floor.

Glass breaks, but I wouldn't consider trading it out for more convenient materials because I like the substance behind it. We received some crystal glasses as a gift years ago. We handle these with care because they are treasures. They remind us of the people who loved us enough to lavish us with these thoughtful gifts. They are special glasses with an intricate cut that reflect the sunlight when they are polished. Just their presence can change the atmosphere of a meal, even making a pizza slice on a paper plate feel like a king's feast because of their beauty.

Relationships are like glass. They can hurt when they are broken. Relationships can shatter into shards and pieces when we are careless, selfish, distracted. But when they are cared for and cleaned with love they are clear and beautiful. Loving relationships bring a sense of joy wherever they are and project brightness onto others nearby. Yes, glass can chip and crack, but did you know it can be repaired? It is costly and it's not easy to find a craftsman who can repair it, but it can be done. A damaged glass can sometimes be restored to its original condition by polishing and grinding it into shape.

Unloving relationships will crack and chip away at each person, but with care and time those imperfections can be polished and mended to make the pieces more beautiful than before. If that friendship, marriage or family relationship was salvaged, we can have a greater sense of appreciation and care for it to hopefully avoid the catastrophe of a full crash and demolition of our relationship in the future.

Cloth products also require care. They get stained and dirty, but can be cleaned and redeemed for future celebrations. I've made cloth napkins from up-cycled cotton plaid shirts. You know, the classic kind with bright colors in soft cotton fabric. After we use them, they just go into the wash with our kitchen towels to be freshened up and used again to brighten up another meal. Whenever I toss something away I think of lost potential and how it could be re-purposed into a treasure. Here are some simple ways to build substance into your home life and trade out the disposables and plastics:

HOME CARE CHOICES

- Treat yourself to cloth napkins instead of disposable, and pack a picnic lunch. Real fibers for a real life. If you have a sewing machine and can make a straight stitch, re-purpose some old shirts into fun plaid napkins that will make any meal a picnic whether you're outside or not. Cut simple squares to the size you'd like and finish the edges.
- Use essential oils as a natural perfume. Did you know the chemical structure of synthetic perfumes is similar to plastic? Be real, choose the natural plant oils for the ultimate sensory experience. Make sure you don't apply citrus oils to sun-exposed skin or you'll be more prone to burning.
- Trade out the plastic shower curtain for a cloth one. It will be easier to clean as you can toss it in the washer and it will last longer too.
- Invest in a glass or stainless steel water bottle. Yes, the glass may be a bit more fragile, but treat it with care and it will last. Having things in our life that endure time and are not

disposable translates to other aspects of our lives as we care for what we have rather than being quick to toss it out.

- Make your food look pretty in stainless steel Bento-Boxes. Asian cultures make elaborate designs with their food in these stackable, stainless steel containers that are a fun trade for plastic or disposable options.
- Buy more clothing made of natural materials like cotton, wool, linen, bamboo, silk and hemp that breathes with our skin. Natural fibers come from living, plant material that coincides with our living selves. If you choose anything in natural fibers, at least make it the pj's you sleep with or bedding you rest on every night.
- Wear shoes made of renewable leather or cloth, using less man-made materials which are often made out of PVC plastic like your shower curtain. Your feet are an entry point into all organs in the body. Keep your feet happy! They'll breathe better, keeping your whole body well. Wool and cotton socks are the best choice for everyday wear. There are some great quality tech-fiber socks for athletics, just give your feet a rest from the man-made fibers each day and go barefoot or wear natural.
- Use a natural rubber yoga mat rather than a PVC one which will off-gas chemicals. That means the chemicals in the mat will degrade over time and emit plastic molecules into the air. Jade Yoga has a nice selection of natural rubber yoga mats.
- Buy some quality re-usable cloth bags to perk up your weekly visits to the grocery store. You'll reduce your plastic footprint and wrap your goods in something that's healthier for people and the planet.
- Find a more natural nail polish. That Poly butyl acrylate is also known as toluene, it's a chemical plasticizer that is in most nail polishes and found to be harmful to humans. Check out http://www.EWG.org to see how your existing products rank for toxicity so you can make better choices.
- Replace traditional feminine care products with bleach-free

and plastic-free options that expose your body to dioxin[151], there are many made with natural cotton. Some women who have switched to re-usable, cloth pads actually experienced less severe monthly symptoms and shorter duration of their period.

Chapter 13: Be Active

GETTING WITH NATURE

"God is always seeking you. Every sunset. Ever clear blue sky. Every ocean wave. The starry host of night. He blankets each new day with the invitation, "I am here."[152] - Louie Giglio

Connecting with nature can awaken our inner desire to understand where we came from. At the root of our beliefs may be the wonder of how we were created. We cannot deny that all things have an origin. In the beginning of time, man walked with bare feet on the dirt and grass. In a broad sense we know that nature is good for us, but scientists are validating it's positive effects on lowering our heart rates, strengthening our immune systems, lowering our stress levels, and improving our outlook on life. Dirt is packed with minerals one good microbes that our hands absorb when we dig into it while gardening. Smelling fresh flowers can elevate our mood, wheatgrass and other growing sprouts are packed with phytonutrients to nourish our bodies. Sunshine on our skin helps our bodies synthesize Vitamin D. We are dependent on nature. The elements of the Earth play a huge role in sustaining us in obvious and subtle ways. Our living, breathing environment brings life to us.

On the flip side we have many man-made obstacles shielding us from the positive benefits of the Earth and Sun on our physical bodies and emotional self. Sunscreens prevent our bodies from absorbing Vitamin D, shoes, asphalt, and buildings put a barrier between us and the earth, wi-fi and cell phone waves fill up our air space and even penetrate into the womb of growing babies.

Entering the natural world connects us with God, our creator. It's grounding, nourishing to our physical and emotional health as well and brings us back to our beginnings. Step into nature to meditate on the wonders He has done and restore your spirit.

> "We don't always need a change; sometimes, we just need a rest, and there is no better place to rest our bodies and our souls than outside" [153]
> - Gary Thomas, Sacred Pathways

Choices "Out There"

- Go outside and get some fresh air to combat indoor air pollution[154]. Breathe deeply.
- Go somewhere quiet that might have an outside view or window. Lowering your emotional and physical stress reduces your cortisol levels. Consistently high cortisol levels (your stress hormones) are hard on the body. When you relax your mind and body, it helps bring your body's chemistry out of the fight/flight/freeze mode and into a state of calm. This is a great skill to teach children who are now living in such a stimulating environment. It's important for all of us to step away into the quiet, but especially children who are still growing and developing[155].
- Grow some sprouts. Not only is it satisfying to watch something grow from a seed, these little seedlings are packed with a multitude of nutrients.
- Celebrate the first day of Summer or any day with a picnic in a park.
- Play with stones. Skip them over the water, embellish them

with an uplifting quote or bible verse, play tic-tac-toe outside with some rocks and chalk. Collect rocks from different geological formations and marvel at the complexity of their creation. Rocks have been around since the beginning of time. They've endured history and symbolize stability. Meditate on God as your rock and your foundation, He doesn't change ever. He just wants to be invited into your life as your center, your solid ground. Psalm 62:7

- Watch ants, bees, birds. They live in community, harmony. Reflect on any harmony in your life, or how you can create more harmony. Even if it's just a new routine like waking up and starting the day with a cup of tea or meeting a friend at the park the same day each week. Healthy routines can bring more harmony into our lives, small steps can add up to greater impact

- Pet a puppy, kitten, or other pet. Visit a Humane Society or pet sit for a friend.

- Climb a tree, or lay down underneath one and gaze at the branches above. Notice the textures and colors in the leaves, the bark, the branches. Trees are always growing and changing. How are you continuing to grow and change?

- Dig in the dirt, plant some seeds or a garden if you have the space and time. Get your hands dirty with rich, black earth and become grounded. Organic soil is rich in immune supporting minerals and nutrients that our skin can absorb[156]. Playing with the earth is also a grounding, it can give us a sense of stability when we're connected with the earth. Tree and plants are rooted into the earth, animals burrow into it, and the soil is full of living microbes that can be good for the human body. Specifically, Bacillus species of bacteria are found in the soil and studied for their benefit in human gut flora as a probiotic source[157].

- Pull some weeds, reflect on the choices you can make in your life. Removing weeds is like pruning away the parts of your life that are not productive or helpful. Rake away the weeds and there is more room for the goodness to grow. Weeds are also like negative viewpoints, attaching themselves to a person's thinking, blocking good ideas from taking root. Weeds (negative thoughts) can sneak into a person's mental garden, but they must be pulled immediately[158]. Manage the garden of your thoughts and choices well and you'll have a flourishing, productive space.

- Plant some flowers, notice their growth at each stage. Nurture the sprouts from seed to flower. Two flowers of the same species look alike, yet there are subtle differences in the petals, the placement of the leave, the shading of the colors. Just like our lives go through tiny changes day by day, all of a sudden, we bloom. Accept yourself in the day to day growth that happens slowly at times, more suddenly at others.
- Play: remember a happy day in your life as a child. Find an activity that just brings pure joy - playing tic-tac-toe with sidewalk chalk on the driveway, hide & seek or tag. Allow yourself to be little again.
- Ride a bike, a kid's bike with a horn and a basket.
- Play on a playground, ride on a swing.
- Dig in the sand. Make it simple with plastic cups or use a bucket of sand toys and make an elaborate castle with a moat. Add water and wash it away. Rebuild as many times as you can while the sun is up.
- Kayak or canoe to explore a river or lake.
- Run barefoot in the grass.
- Hike in a nearby park that you haven't discovered yet. Change it up and walk at night with a flashlight or headlamp.
- Turn the lights off, go outside and watch the stars.
- Sleep under the stars.

"There is something of the divine mystery in everything that exists. We can see it sparkle in a sunflower or a poppy. We sense more of this unfathomable mystery in a butterfly that flutters from a twig-or in a goldfish swimming in a bowl. But we are closest to God in our own soul. Only there can we become one with the great mystery of life." [159]

- Jostein Gaarder

Chapter 14: Be Safe

FINDING WHAT IS SAFE AND SECURE FOR YOU

Being able to secure and protect ourselves depends on our health and well-being physically and emotionally. If you're not in a stable situation, you will need to make choices and form habits that bring some sense of security until things resolve. These baby steps can help re-build awareness and your sense of safety over time, ministering to your true needs in a dysfunctional situation. However, they're not a replacement for poor choices which may be compounding your distress.

Safety is essential to our physical, emotional and spiritual well-being. If we don't feel safe, we cannot fully live. When you find moments that you feel safe, hold on to them, remember them! Our feelings of safety are also often closely linked with how much rest we're giving ourselves and stillness to understand our thoughts and emotions, have time to reflect and pray for insight. When we're overtired, we're more vulnerable to misunderstanding situations or people which can make us feel unsafe.

Use these prompts to take responsibility for your own healing and bring yourself into safety when you can. To get the most out of these steps in the long run, it will help to turn away from as many destructive behaviors or situations as you can.

REST gives us space to recover our strength after trauma. It gives us the space to connect our physical body with our emotions, mind and our spirit. This REST prompt can be a part of your Sabbath each day or week.

Remove yourself physically & emotionally from unhealthy situations.

Embrace the present moment - focus on your breath patterns, not looking at the past or worrying about the future. Just focusing on your breath is a simple way to practice being present.

Stretch your physical body through movement, your mind as you observe your body, meditate and pray through the exercise. When you experience discomfort in your physical body, invite your emotions and spirit into the practice to reflect on other aspects of your life that you might feel stretched. Apply the stretching techniques you learned from Chapter 8.

Teach your mind and body to better understand yourself and your creator as you draw wisdom from Him. This is a place you can learn to self-regulate and move your body responses out of habitual reactions and into more controlled, intentional direction. Slowing down our body through yoga allows the best of us to emerge through self-awareness, acceptance and adjustment to the discoveries we encounter through God's grace.

"Having hope will give you courage. You will be protected and will
rest in safety"
- Job 11:18

- Use a weighted blanket. The heaviness of a weighted
  blanket gives us the same perceptions as receiving a hug.
  Did you know scientists have actually determined that each
  of us needs at least eight hugs a day to be healthy?[160]

We need 4 hugs a day for survival.
We need 8 hugs a day for maintenance.
We need 12 hugs a day for growth
- Virginia Satir, Psychotherapist

- Keep something familiar, safe with you: a small piece of
  fabric, or familiar scent in an essential oil roll-on bottle.
  Memorize a comforting scripture or quote when you hold
  onto this item. This connection will begin to form re-wiring
  in your brain to connect your thoughts with your actions.
  Eventually, you may be able to eliminate the object but
  continue to hold onto your positive thoughts or affirmations
  in faith. The goal is not to find an object to latch onto but
  to eventually free ourselves of earthly items that we feel we
  need for long-term security. As our confidence grows and
  healing happens inside of us we rely less on the "earthly"
  for true support.
- Visualize your safe place: be in the quiet and think of
  sights, sounds, smells, textures, and tastes from a place that
  makes you happy. It could be a time and place from your

childhood, a destination from a vacation. Wherever that space is, close your eyes and fully immerse yourself in the memory of it. Recall as many details as you can to almost transport yourself back to that place in time. Take as much time as you like for this activity, or just a few minutes. Anyway you practice it can help bring you into a sense of security and relief from the daily stressors of life.

- Build rest time into each day and week so you can recover your physical bodies from work, renew your minds from emotional stress and connect your spirit in faith. When we carve out time each day, even 15 minutes, for quiet and rest it creates a healthy foundation for self-care.
- Make a list of good friends. Star the ones who you feel you can share pieces of your life and who have shared with you pieces of their life. For each friend, think of one thing you can do to deepen the friendship and plan a time to do that.
- Rearrange your closet so your most comfortable and favorite clothes are all in one spot. Find and add one new thing every few months.
- Keep a list of activities that you can do when you feel anxious so that you're prepared when the time comes to replace or manage those feelings with healthy outlets.
- Re-do or create any photo albums that remind you of the blessings in your life. Create a wall for framed pictures in your home.
- Find scriptures (yourself, or ask a believing friend) that point to God's promises and love. Keep them in a prominent place such as in your purse, on the bathroom mirror, in frames around the house.
- Keep a CD or digital storage of your favorite songs that bring you peace.
- Write yourself an empowering letter for a future date or anniversary. Mark your calendar to remind you to read it.
- Serve the more vulnerable in your community: the elderly, homeless, unwed mothers, women's shelter. It may be a

meal, letter, game night, or something simple and gentle. Through serving, we find strength and confidence that love and care are abundant within us.

PART THREE TAKEAWAYS

We have so many choices in how we can care for ourselves and the environment in which we live. In the various lists we've explored in this section, we've found that sometimes the best choices aren't always the most advertised or easiest to find. I encourage you to pick one or two categories and make a plan to implement a few new choices. The three considerations below will help you to make the changes a reality:

1. **Distractions** The internet is flooded with marketing campaigns for personal care items, recipes and exercise tips. Consider where you are bombarded with information and look at unsubscribing to some newsletters or unfollowing pages to free up your social media feeds. Look at real books as resources because they give you the space to think and read and consider ways to apply information. Not all information and sources can be trusted. Be wary of any marketing campaigns that give you limited time to make decisions for purchases. If anyone is pressuring you to make a purchase immediately, walk away for a couple of days and take time to think about it. Distractions in our life make us vulnerable to making poor decisions in any situation. The better you understand yourself, motives and priorities, the less distractions will sway you from those core beliefs. When have you gotten caught up in marketing hype? Have you ever felt buyer's remorse? How long did it take to surface? Write any notes below of distractions you are aware of and how you could manage them.

2. **Direction** Discovering some new habits that keep us on track with our goals is invaluable. Equally valuable is surrounding

ourselves with like-minded individuals who have similar goals. There are many local clubs, organizations or church groups that have small communities we can tap into that encourage us to keep making positive and intelligent choices. Re-write your mission statement here to affirm your choices.

3. **Decisions** Forming new habits and making choices that are unfamiliar to us takes discipline and perseverance. The effort is worth it! By now, hopefully you are experiencing better insight into your life and where you'd like to make positive changes. Now is the time you can start making some intentional choices. Highlight, check off boxes, write notes in the margins next to the ideas that jump out at you. What has gotten your attention? Start with some of those choices first. Get those decisions on your calendar, on your grocery list, and in that short to-do list you make each morning. As you fit them into your daily routines they will become more familiar and eventually won't feel as awkward. It might help to keep a journal of your experiences so you can understand better what might be working. And is there someone who can hold you accountable for your new choices? Does your calendar align with your goals? What decisions would you like to stick with in the coming month? Write them here.

Goal	Choice	Notes
Ex: Drink less caffeine	Trade out 1 coffee a day for water	
	Find natural sources of energy	

COMMUNITY
CONNECTIONS

Extending Beyond Ourselves
to
Connect In Community
Develop our Sense of Purpose & Value

At the core of relationship building and volunteering/ giving back is building a sense of community. God encouraged His people to meet together regularly because He knew they needed each other. The power of association offers so much to the dynamics of our lives. If we hang around people who complain about jobs and spouses, it won't be long before we hate our job and think we have a slug for a spouse. The stress of those kinds of thoughts always manifests itself in health and overall attitude. But do things with people who realize that no matter what task they are doing, they are going to do it for the glory of God and you are on a mission! Be in regular conversation with others who speak blessings over their spouse and do things to love and serve and soon you'll be energized to make that relationship better than you ever thought it could be.

Chapter 15: Giving Back

"Your love has given me great joy and encouragement, because you have refreshed the hearts of the Lord's people" Philemon 1:7

There are practical reasons for community such as work tasks and committees, but we also need to build in time with others for for emotional and spiritual support. Touching the theme again that we are mind, body and spirit, let's explore how the power of community brings wholeness and health.

We can support each other with physical needs like making a meal for a friend, encouraging one another, and praying with each other to keep us connected spiritually. Any opportunity to volunteer holds the potential to be a community building experience. Obviously, any ongoing volunteering in the same place will impact members in a different way than a one-time event. We all need to be a part of a community, and our roles in a healthy community will fluctuate from giver to receiver. Each of us is in different seasons of our life and you'll get the most out of community building if you have a good understanding what season you're in.

Dynamics That Affect Our Place In Any Community:

- Our innate sense of wanting to belong
- Desires to be accepted and loved through authentic connections
- Our present capability to give & receive
- Health of our soul in forming safe boundaries = avoiding
- Co-Dependency, prioritizing and gauging commitment
- Building community through healthy habits
- Discovering community building activities that foster authentic relationships Working with others on common mission

Not everyone is in a position to give in their current season of life, but everyone has a need to be part of a community. I've been in many seasons of life where I had to sit on the sidelines or pull back from serving because it was not the right time. When my children were little, we weren't as portable as some families are today and would get overwhelmed if there were too many scheduled activities and play dates. I craved some routine in their lives and that limited what I could accomplish outside our home. In those seasons, social media was a great tool to keep me connected with other stay at home moms who craved connection with other adults. This season of parenting left me with limited opportunities to serve, but I did what I could at the time. Most often I'd bring healthy meals to moms who just had a baby, or served in classrooms that my kids were in.

One season surprised me and brought me great growth personally and spiritually. When I was newer to faith, I felt God nudging me to be involved in some way in church even thought I felt totally inadequate to serve. When my first boy was just four years-old, I stepped in to help teach little ones about God in small worship sessions. It was awkward at first because I felt like a toddler in my own faith, but this was just were God wanted me to be. I served alongside Teresa, a mother of some older kids, but her youngest was the same age as my oldest. During that year of serving and teaching, thankfully with the help of a curriculum, I was blessed to observe Teresa and her loving care for each of the children. I learned so many lessons myself, but picked up Teresa as a mentor, helping me become a better parent, wife and person. To this day, I continue to remember the way she simply loved those children through teaching.

That is what I gained!

But what I offered also blessed me. Her modeling was inspiration to me to step up and serve with little children in my own church, singing and teaching them in faith. Now I am not a professional singer or musician at all, but my heart is to love these children and pass on a love of learning and new discovery that they matter. I just offered up my time and care and God used it to bless the children. I also grew in my own faith as I taught and cared for the kids in a volunteer situation. I was reading and learning about the same things as they were. Simple truths in a clear way. When you step up to serve others it returns back to you in a fulfillment that takes the focus off of yourself, including worldly pressures, our own battles and insecurities, even if only for an hour.

I grew up in a home with some out of balance serving perspectives. I love my mom and the way she raised me, she is a survivor and peacemaker with a servant heart, but sometimes to the extent that she puts her own needs on the back burner. I believe this influence is from her generation to serve others so deeply. It's a character trait that can provide a sense of community and support as long as it's not taken advantage of. I've experienced this time and again in my own life that where one is willing to give, there are some in a habit of always receiving, which can fuel a dysfunctional, co-dependent relationship. It's taken a long time to re-work those habits, some of which I fall back into at time because of the familiarity of them.

Learn to say "no" to the good things so you can say "yes" to the greater!

Months prior to writing this book, the busy-ness crept back into my schedule as I slowly said "yes" to a few too many opportunities to give. It was painful to have to prune away those activities as I realized my bucket was going to be empty pretty quickly if I continued on the path I was headed. Building boundaries can feel awkward if we're not used to having them, but they are necessary in living a healthy emotional life and creating lasting friendships. Practice setting safe boundaries with small decisions like those listed here so that you build confidence in creating boundaries within more complex situations.

If you are suffering from caregiver burnout, this probably isn't the best place to focus your self-care unless it energizes you. For example, if you're a counselor for abused women, but you love animals and have enjoyed serving at a local animal shelter on your days off. This is great! But serving more time at a women's shelter on the weekend with the same type of clients you're with during business hours might not feel like you have a break from work. Or, maybe you're already taking care of elderly parents as part of the 'Sandwich Generation'. You're not likely to spend your free time volunteering at a nursing home to energize yourself, right? Remember to give yourself the oxygen first…..variety is good in these situations. Effective self-care involves having a better understanding of your energy levels, current responsibilities and nurturing your mind, body and spirit. Choose your volunteer work to compliment the other aspects of your life rather than activities that compete with your energy.

Know your limits and capacity to give back, and be open to being on the receiving end of building community. Different seasons of life allow you to offer varying levels of commitment. If the concept of volunteering is new to you or you're going through therapy yourself, start small. Often the best way to grow in confidence in ourselves is to help someone else in greater need, but make sure it isn't letting you fall into old habits of dysfunction like people pleasing or seeking affirmation for the wrong reasons.

In many situations, the best gift you can give is commitment. It may feel vulnerable to commit to it a set time or task, but those volunteer relationships are invaluable to those you're helping and it will bless your spirit. You'll feel more satisfaction and peace when you see relationship build over time. If you are not in a season that you feel you can give, let that go. Remember, part of honoring your self is recognizing your limits physically, emotionally and spiritually. There are many communities you can become a part of, if you are limited with drive time or location, look at opportunities to stay in connection with others online.

Connecting as a Volunteer:

- Volunteer at a local food pantry.
- Tutor at-risk or struggling kids after school.
- Serve home-cooked meals at a local hospital for long term patients or home-bound elderly.
- Read stories to kids or the elderly in a nursing home,

- Hold babies in the hospital when parents can't be with them.
- Make cookies for a local fire or police department and send along a thank you note for their work to keep our community safe.
- Make a meal for an expectant mom, love on her and support her in growing this amazing miracle.
- Leave a gift card for the next person in line at the coffee shop.
- Shovel a neighbor's sidewalk or help them with yard work.
- Share a meal with someone whenever you can - extend an invitation to others and receive it when it's offered.
- Build someone up online at least once every time you are on social media. If someone is on your mind, tell them.

Start small and fit the giving to your current season of life. It is not your job to save the world! What matters is your heart in giving. If this is not your season to extend care, stepping back from a volunteer opportunity will give someone else a chance to step in.

"The eye is the lamp of the body. If your eyes are healthy, your whole body will be full of light." Matthew 6:22

At first glance this verse might seem to be literally about what we see, which is important. When we see beautiful things physically, emotionally, spiritually, it gives us a lift in our spirit that others can detect. But the key word in this verse is "healthy". This is not healthy in the sense that our modern culture defined, such as physically, but it refers to a sense of our spirit or nature. The word healthy in this verse is a heart condition, such as our motives. When we give for the right reasons at the right time, we will be a light in the world. Giving out of unmet needs, to feel accepted, or for tendencies to manipulate others is formed out of co-dependency and can be hurtful to the giver and the receiver. I include this chapter as a step for those who are ready to serve from your heart with pure intentions, to give freely without accepting anything in return. This is the place of light that we can be. It doesn't have to be some grandiose act of heroism, rather the small acts of kindness we can do in the everyday moments of our lives that will create wholeness in our mind, body and spirit.

Chapter 16: Building Relationships Within a Community

The moment we begin to see accept our authentic selves is the place we can meet others in genuine community.

Doing life with others, whether serving together, studying together or just having fellowship with each other is where relationships can flourish. Many people haven't grown up with healthy role-models of what it looks like to engage in life-giving relationships. We have many opportunities to grow closer with others if we let down our walls and look at differences as a way to strengthen our inter-relational skills rather than as an excuse to avoid someone different from us. Surrounding ourselves with a variety of personalities and those with varying interests from ourselves can improve our communication skills, give us patience in understanding those with other viewpoints than our own, and give us insight to how other's process information. We can learn a great deal about ourselves and others when we interact with those different than ourselves. Look at the communities you're already involved in, or seek out groups in your church or community as a safe place to begin connecting with others if you aren't connected yet.

Here are 10 specific activities you could do with a group on a weekly or monthly basis. Use these activity prompts as a springboard to deeper conversations about the discussion points and as a tool to building a stronger community. Healthy communities extend grace, acceptance, loyalty and encouragement no matter where you are in your journey.

Connecting for Relationship

- Start a book study in your neighborhood or with a group of friends.
- Create a list of people you could call, maybe one a week, with the purpose of connecting on an encouraging and supportive level.

- Make a plan to get out of the house one day a week or month to go meet new people or do a new thing.

- Join a Bible study through your church.
- Join a club/business that meets regularly for personal development.
- Drop letters and cards in the mail frequently to friends and family, sharing your news and asking theirs.

- Go for a walk in the neighborhood and when you see others, make a point to wave and say hello. Try to engage others in even a simple conversation. Sometimes you meet people who need more connecting!

- Join a support group through a hospital or church or community organization that shares a concern or struggle you have.

- Keep up on local festivals, art shows, musicals or plays and attend when you can.

- Host a pie-making contest or a chili contest at work, in the neighborhood or through a cause-driven organization.

"You are the light of the world—like a city on a hilltop that cannot be hidden. No one lights a lamp and then puts it under a basket. Instead, a lamp is placed on a stand, where it gives light to everyone in the house. In the same way, let your good deeds shine out for all to see, so that everyone will praise your heavenly Father.
Matthew 5:13-16

God uses each of us to bring love, light and grace to one another. Step into the gap and multiply His work.

Chapter 17: Our Final Connection

Integrating and honoring our mind, body and spirit as elements that work together gives us the confidence and courage to live our lives with intention. And inviting God into every aspect of our life can be the compass that guides us in each and every decision you make, whether we bump a failure or skip into a success. With God guiding the process, we can experience the grace, compassion and abundance that was planned for us long before we were born. There is a plan and a purpose for your life, one that is filled with abundance and joy! The changes won't always be easy, but be brave! You will have so much to discover and so much to be proud of!

"Life cannot be satisfied when it is lived out as a consuming entity. When it is filled by that which satisfies a hunger that is both physical and spiritual in a mutuality that sustains both without volition of either, only then can life be truly fulfilling."
Ravi Zacharias

As I conclude this map, a guide for treating your body as a temple of the Holy Spirit, I see the importance of emphasizing the most important relationship you can choose to be a part of. We have found little bits of comfort and encouragement all along in/on this Two inches of Wool, but there is one last connection with which I wish to leave you. Throughout the Bible, the One True God is shown in relationship with his people symbolically as a shepherd is to his sheep. While historical accounts of a shepherd in Biblical times are not directly relevant to our modern lives, the relationships they demonstrate cross all barriers of time. A kind shepherd has a deep love for his sheep for many reasons, and a shepherd will sacrifice many things for the protection of his flock. You see, his flock wasn't just a source of livelihood because of the wool they provide, although the wool was a great blessing. A shepherd raises most of his sheep from birth, and they are his closest family. He tends them when they are sick, rescues them when they are troubled and cares for them every day as he gently guides them with his rod. He loves to be with them. Sheep get startled easily and the shepherd's constant presence calms their anxious hearts as he guides them along rolling and rocky hills. The nature of a shepherd is to watch over every one of his sheep as a valued treasure, to care for it, lead it to green pastures for grazing and to clean waters for thirst. A shepherd protects his sheep from enemies and guides his sheep to rest each day. He will search the world over for one that is lost. In fact, the shepherd sees the lost sheep as even more valuable as the others because of his desire to restore it to it's safe place in the flock. The shepherd will stop at nothing to find that little lost one and bring it back to care for it once again.

Do you long to be known? To be accepted and loved in a way like you've never felt before? To be guided in all that you do, to nourish your body, restore your soul and find complete rest? Jesus was often referred to as the Good Shepherd because of all these ways He cares for us if we allow Him to and He extends the invitation to you to join His flock. My prayer is that as you read about the possibilities of a deep, loving relationship with Jesus that you would consider his love for you as a shepherd loves his sheep.

Jesus is always here. His gracious, gentle, kind Spirit wants to share your life. You can come to the place in your heart where you know you really do belong to Him. You can see He cares for you. You can be His, the invitation is always there for you on your Two Inches of Wool.

RESOURCES

Community Building Activities

15 Staples For Natural Cooking

15 Beauty Foods

15 Foods To Support Liver and Kidney Health

15 Hidden Sources of Corn

Simple Recipes

15 Natural Resources For Home and Personal Care

15 Helps For Sleep

15 Essential Oils and Their Uses

15 Essential Oils For Liver and Kidney Health

10 Common Mistakes EO Users Make

Home Spa Recipes

Resources for Supplies and Healthy Foods

National Hotlines

Scriptures

Community Building Activities

1. Share a Meal: Make a pot of Immune Building soup together. Everyone can bring a vegetable, chop them together and have your discussion as the soup cooks. Discussion focus: What are the unique qualities of each person, your "Super Power"? We all have different gifts, interests and experiences. Have each person share a strength of theirs and how they can use that to bless others. Encourage others to offer ideas of how that strength can be used for good. Talk about a character trait you'd like to develop and hold each other accountable: write it down and encourage each other to keep it up. Some character traits: Consistent, Courageous, Compassionate, Cooperative, Creative, Detailed, Determined, Discerning, Gentle, Generous, Flexible, Observant, Optimistic, Patient, Peaceful, Perseverant, Resourceful. How can we use our gift to encourage others?

Scripture Focus: Hebrews 10:24-25 "Let's consider how we can spur one another on toward love and good deeds, not giving up meeting together, as some are in the habit of doing, but encouraging one another-all the more as you see the day coming."

2. Game Night: Pick a few games to play, keep it simple with a deck of cards or board games. Have guests bring their own favorite if they have one, if you have a non-profit partner see if they have resources to supply some. Discussion: Talk about any happy memories you might have, no matter how small. Share with friends something that brings a smile to your face whenever you think of it. This might become your "safe place". If someone in your group is struggling with finding a positive memory, be patient with them. Building healthy community with others involves being vulnerable which can be very difficult for many people. If someone doesn't want to share a personal experience, offer an option to share your favorite flavor of ice cream or food.

Scripture focus Romans 15:32 So that by God's will I may come to you with joy and be refreshed together with you.

3. Spa Night: Pick a DIY project or two and make them together. Essential oil Body Spray and a Simple Lip Balm are easy to make. (See Directions In Spa Recipes Section) Discussion focus: Talk about real beauty. How do you define it? How do you feel pressured to define it? Talk about God's definition of beauty and how you can encourage each other in a healthy body image.

Scripture focus 1 Peter 3:3-4 "Your beauty should be that of your inner self, the unfading beauty of a gentle and quiet spirit, which is of great worth in God's sight."

4. Art Night: Create an art project: painting, journaling or whatever your group decides on. Discussion focus: You are a Masterpiece! What are dreams you have for your life? Incorporate them into your art project as inspiration to reach for your dreams! Encourage each other and find something positive to say about each person and their work of art.

Scripture focus Ephesians 2:10 "For you are God's workmanship, created in Christ Jesus to do good works, which He prepared in advance for you to do."

5. Hiking, Nature Walk: Visit a local park, beach, or nature preserve, anywhere you can be outdoors and enjoy peace and quiet. Focus on being still, being comfortable with silence and yourself. Have a discussion afterwards of how you felt doing this. Talk about what you are observing inside yourself and your surroundings. Journal or draw out your thoughts.

Scripture focus Jeremiah 17:10 & Romans 8:27. "He who searches our hearts knows the mind of the Spirit, because the Spirit intercedes for us according to God's will.

6. Grow a garden or plant some flowers: Each person can plant their own seeds in a pot, make it a tiny herb garden or flowers. Moisten the soil and cover the pot with plastic wrap to seal in moisture. For more immediate results, take a flat of seedlings and divide them up among guests. Each guest will get a small pot with a young plant they can care for and watch grow. **Discussion focus:** We are all growing in some way, what are some choices we can make in our life that will keep us growing in the right direction and nurture those seedlings? Talk about obstacles to growth, encourage guests to problem solve with each other to find solutions for overcoming challenges to personal growth.

Scripture focus Matthew 17:20 "If you have faith as small as a mustard seed, you can say to this mountain, 'Move from here to there' and it will move. Nothing will be impossible for you."

7. Vision Boarding Snack Buffet: Vision boarding is a business tool that helps brainstorm ideas for a project or person. It can also be a personal tool in discovering your personal strengths, weaknesses, dreams and goal-setting. Each guest can bring different vegetables, dips, nuts, fresh herbs, seeds, or embellishments for an hors d'ovures buffet. The goal is to have a variety of colors, flavors, and textures that guests can pick from. Place ingredients on decorative plates and arrange them in an interesting way that is visually appealing. If you want, choose a theme like a country and focus on foods and decorations that represent that place. French cheeses, Mexican chiles, Tropical island. Invite guests to create colorful and creative arrangements with their ingredients that are pleasing to the eye. This artistic expression will open up creativity in your vision boarding activity that will encourage individual expression.

Buffet ideas

- Vegetables: chopped bell peppers, shredded carrots, small broccoli spears, thin-sliced cucumbers, fresh sprouts, water chestnuts, cherry tomatoes sliced in half
- Fruits: tiny apple wedges, pomegranates seeds, strawberry slices,
- Seeds: Sunflower seeds, chia seeds, pumpkin seeds
- Cheeses: small wedges, thin slices, soft brie, aged cheddar, swiss, gouda, fresh mozzarella
- Fresh herbs: chopped basil, tarragon leaves, dill sprigs, chives in 1-inch strips, rosemary leaves, cilantro leaves
- Crackers & bread: Gluten free crackers (Mary's Gone Crackers are made with colorful seeds), textured crackers, small bread slices
- Spreads: Guacamole, hummus, artichoke dip, cream cheese.

Discussion focus: Understanding where you are going will determine the path you will go. Use this vision boarding activity to decide with intention what direction you want to head. What is your vision led with? Passion for a cause? Faith? Money? Look back on your "Why" exercise and decide if your "vision" could use some editing. Discuss obstacles to reaching that vision, acknowledging if it needs revision so you can re-set your course. It's easy to get off the path we intend just because of the nature of our society, filled with distractions. Use this vision board activity to build intention into your goal-setting, personal mission statement and desires to find wholeness in your mind, body and spirit.

Scripture focus Proverbs 20:5 " The purposes of a man's heart are deep waters, but a man of understanding draws them out."

8. Yoga - Relaxation Class : Have a yoga session or simple stretch session and focus on stress management skills as well as self-awareness of your physical body. Don't be surprised if some emotions open up. As you stretch your physical body, consider how you are being stretched in other areas of your life: relationships, personal goals, emotional healing and spiritual growth. **Discussion focus:** Talk about where you feel stretched in your life. How can you encourage others in your group to embrace positive changes and let go of harmful influences?

Scripture focus Psalm 46:1-7 "God is our refuge and our strength, a great help in times of distress."

9. Puzzle Challenge: Bring in different puzzles, a large one for everyone to work on together or several small. If you have the choice, bring in puzzles that are colorful with positive and inspiring images. Have guests build puzzles during your gathering. **Discussion focus:** We are all interconnected, we make a picture of wholeness. All parts belong to each other and need the others to make a completed project. Ask guests to talk about how they see each other fitting in to the community. How do they see choices in their lives affecting their mind, body and spirit? Share some good examples of what choices may have a positive impact on all areas of our life.

Scripture focus 1 Corinthians 12:12-27

10. April Fools Foods Night: Make one dish or have several people bring in a different "dish" to pass. These should be a dish that looks like one thing but are another. Talk about how outward appearances can be deceptive. How can we live more authentic lives with ourselves and others?

Cracked Egg Cupcakes

http://www.yummly.co/recipe/Cracked-Egg-April-Fool_s-Cupcakes-1037828?prm-v1

Dessert Taco Salad

http://www.cakecentral.com/gallery/i/1629965/april-fools-taco-salad

Cheese Carrots & Crackers

https://shewearsmanyhats.com/cheese-carrots/

Apple French Fries

http://www.food.com/recipe/april-fools-day-fooled-ya-french-fries-159047

Spaghetti Cupcakes

http://blog.uniquelygrace.com/2011_03_27_archive.html

Scripture focus 1 John 3:18 "Let's not merely say that we love each other; let us show the truth by our actions." (NLT)

11. Gratitude Gathering: Supply thank you cards or blank cards and stamping, art or drawing supplies for guests to make their own thank you cards. Each person can write out one or several thank you cards to someone in their life they appreciate. Include stamps so they can be mailed by snail mail. **Discussion focus:** Giving Thanks for the people in your life, share something positive someone has done in your life and how it inspired you.

Scripture focus: 1 Thessalonians 5:18 "Give thanks in every circumstance"

12. Pottery Studio: Visit a pottery studio where you can form a clay pot, cup or other creation. Enjoy how different everyone's creations are, each unique in their own ways. Discuss ways that you are all changing or would like to change, exchanging ideas of what habits or qualities are easier to change and which ones are more difficult. Are there any behaviors that might be more permanent or others which might be more flexible to form to healthier ways?

Scripture focus Isaiah 64:8 "O Lord, you are our Father. We are the clay, you are the potter; we are all the work of your hand."

13. Go On A Picnic: Have everyone bring a different finger food, one that transports easily and can be shared. Someone can be in charge of blankets or tablecloth and others the meal specifics. The focus can be on working together, we are all the body with many parts and gifts that complement the others. We are all part of community. Here are some ideas:

- Fruit kabobs
- Sliced veggies & dip
- Cubed cheeses on toothpicks
- Crackers, Gluten-Free options
- Cubed chicken chunks
- Bottled water, juice or tea
- Gluten-free dessert (Recipe ideas in back)
- Plates, napkins, utensils
- Blankets, Tablecloth or Sheet to put on the ground or on a picnic table

Scripture focus Colossians 3:14-15 "Above all, clothe yourselves with love which binds us together in perfect harmony."

14. Serve Together at a local shelter, hospital, food pantry or other organization in need in your area. If you are able, make it a regular outing and opportunity for your group to get to know others in the organization.

Scripture focus 1 Peter "Each of you should use whatever gift you have received to serve others".

15. Have a Tea Party (based on Dannah Gresh Secret Keeper Girl Study). Bring out the real china and celebrate your real, authentic beauty. Enjoy time together as friends and just take time to talk and listen to each other. Discussion points: What makes you feel beautiful? Celebrate the beauty in each person of your gathering. Talk about how we can treasure relationships and value each other. Work through difficulties instead of being quick to throw away a friendship (like a disposable cup). Do you know the process it takes to make a porcelain tea cup? True porcelain has a glass-like appearance, a beauty that has been valued and sought after for centuries. The porcelain materials are ground up, smashed, thrown down, and finally pressed into shape. They are fired a first time to vaporize impurities and then covered with a glaze. The materials used for the glaze go through a meticulous preparation to remove contaminants that might take away from the beauty of the cup. The porcelain is fired in a kiln again at temperatures reaching 2,650 degrees Fahrenheit![161] This firing is done to bond all the precious ingredients together for an exquisite piece of porcelain that is not only beautiful, it is strong. Practice speaking words that build other's up and celebrate the gifts each person has. Our society may send messages that don't always bring life to relationships and may tempt us to "throw away" a person or treat them as disposable out of convenience, low self-esteem or competitive spirit. Take time to affirm the value of each person and how they can bless others with their life.

Scripture focus: Isaiah 43:2 "When you go through deep waters, I will be with you. When you go through the rivers of difficulty, you will not be overwhelmed; when you walk through fire of oppression you will not be burned up; the flames will not consume you." (NLT & ESV versions)

16. Worship Together: Talk about your faith and beliefs with each other in a respectful manner. Consider visiting each other's places of worship and talk about the messages, thoughts or impressions (with care) afterwards. This activity will most likely challenge you to consider other's identities apart from their beliefs, priorities and faith, especially if they are different from your own. A healthy perspective is to focus on the positive and make sure you frame questions in a positive light. It might help to just make an observation: "I noticed during the service we did _____, what is the meaning behind this?" Be careful how you share your feelings and make sure to use perspectives such as "I felt", "I observed", "I noticed" rather than "you should", "you shouldn't", or hurtful words like "that's weird, dumb, stupid. Think of how you might want someone to speak it before you say it out loud, pausing before you talk. It's normal to feel a little uncomfortable when you begin talking about personal ideas and beliefs, but the effort will be worth it in deeper connections with others when it's carried out with kindness and respect.

Scripture focus: Romans 12:9-13 "Love must be sincere. Hate what is evil; cling to what is good. Be devoted to one another in brotherly love. Honor one another above yourselves. Never be lacking in zeal, but keep your spiritual fervor, serving the Lord. Be joyful in hope, patient in affliction, faithful in prayer. Share with God's people who are in need. Practice hospitality.

SIMPLE RECIPES

Veggie Immune Soup

Roasted Butternut Squash Soup

Chicken Bone Broth

Basic Smoothie

Turmeric Tea: Golden Milk

Overnight Oatmeal

Fermented Veggies

Carrot & Walnut Salad

Roasted-Grilled Veggies

Basic Vinaigrette

Grilled Tarragon Chicken: Meat Marinade

Pad Thai

Coconut-flour brownies Chia Seed pudding

No Bake Truffles & Paleo Granola

Almond Flour Muffins

Caramel No-Bake Pumpkin Seed Bars

Veggie Immune Soup

Makes 6 servings

Soup is soul food. It's also super easy to make your own with flavors you love. All vegetables are packed with antioxidants and immune supporting nutrients. This recipe can be customized with other vegetables you might have on hand, although the Shitake mushrooms and Astragalus are the ingredients that give it the immune-building power. Astragalus is an ingredient some health food stores carry in their bulk spice section and of course you can find it online at many natural food and herbal shops like Mountain Rose Naturals. **bit.ly/ImmuneSoup**

1 large onion

3 cloves garlic minced

2 T olive oil

4-5 Astragalus sticks (look like tongue depressors)

2 parsnips, chopped

1 C each celery and green beans, chopped

2 C carrots, chopped

2 large potatoes, chopped

2 fresh Shitake mushrooms, or 1-2 dried

Flavoring herbs to taste, 1-2 Tablespoons fresh chopped (basil, tarragon, parsley, oregano)

Saute onion & garlic in oil. Add 8 C pure water and bring to a boil. Add vegetables and simmer, covered 1 hour. Add herbs last 10 minutes. Strain out Astragalus & serve. 6 servings.

Roasted Butternut Squash Soup

2 T organic butter

2 T Extra Virgin Olive oil, cold pressed & organic (EVO)

2 small organic onions, diced

3 large cloves organic garlic

2 oz. organic cream cheese

Pinch of sea salt

Fresh ground pepper to taste

2 lbs steamed butternut squash, peeled and cubed

6 T organic white Miso dissolved in 4 C purified water

2 drops food grade oregano essential oil

1 drop food grade lemon essential oil

Peel and seed the butternut squash. Place on a cookie sheet lined with parchment paper and drizzle with 1 tablespoon of olive oil.

Roast in a 350 degree oven for 30-40 minutes until tender. A fork inserted into squash should pierce in smoothly. Put this aside. **bit.ly/ButternutSquashSOUP**

Heat a 4 quart saucepan over medium heat. When hot, add butter and olive oil. When the butter is melted, add onions and saute' for 1-2 minutes until they are soft. Add garlic and cream cheese. Heat until the cream cheese is melted, adding sea salt and pepper to taste.

Add squash to mixture and sauce 1-2 minutes. Add miso broth and bring mixture to a boil. Allow to cool, then spoon out 1/2 the mixture into a blender and blend until smooth. Return mixture to the saucepan.

Add essential oils last and allow the soup to simmer for 5 minutes. Garnish with whole grain or gluten free croutons, shredded carrots or fresh oregano.

- Make sure you only use essential oils labeled as dietary supplements that are safe for ingestion.
- What is MISO? Miso is a fermented soy product that is superior to tofu which still contains phytic acid which blocks the absorption of many essential nutrients. Miso is rich in Omega-3 fatty acids and a complete protein meant to be ingested in small amounts. It gives the soup a rich, savory flavor.

Chicken Bone Broth

Makes 3-4 quarts

This nourishing broth is simple to make and doesn't have all the artificial flavorings of store bought. This is a staple in our family and we make a batch every week during the Fall and Winter to use as a base for soups, cooking rice and vegetables or just on it's own to nurture someone who's under the weather. It's great for hydration when someone is recovering from a cold. **bit.ly/SimpleBoneBroth**

(Tip: save your cooked chicken bones in a ziplock freezer bag until you have enough to make a large pot of broth, also save your organic vegetable clippings - onions, carrots, celery, potatoes, in a ziplock bag in your freezer. When you make your bone broth, toss in a few handfuls of the clippings to add some extra flavor and nutrients)

1 whole chicken, raw or chicken bones from a cooked bird

Enough water to cover the chicken (4-6 quarts for just bones, 8-10 quarts for a larger, whole bird)

1 Small onion, chopped (if you're not using vegetable clippings)

Cover chicken or bones with purified water. Simmer 18-24 hours. If you are using a whole, raw chicken, you can remove much of the meat after 2-3 hours or until it is cooked through and use for another meal.

If you are using a stove burner, cook for 10-12 hours one day, refrigerate and then continue cooking a second day for 10-12 hours. Alternatively, you may use a slow cooker, just make sure your cooker's ceramic dish is lead-free.

Allow the broth to cool slightly and then use immediately, freeze in individual ice cube trays for future use or refrigerate for up to 3 days.

Basic Smoothies

Fruits smoothie vs Veggie smoothie: keep fruit and vegetables separate to avoid stress on the digestive tract:

bit.ly/PurePopsicles

Fruit smoothie: 1/2 C frozen berries, 1/2 C water, herbal tea or coconut water

Veggie smoothie: 1 C greens (spinach, parsley or baby kale), 1/2 avocado, 1/2 cucumber, 1/2 C water or coconut water.

Optional Add-ins: 1 scoop of protein powder or 1 tsp chia seeds

Combine ingredients in a blender. If using fresh produce, add a few ice cubes to thicken.

Turmeric Tea - Golden Milk

Turmeric Tea is a traditional India drink. The recipe can vary from family to family depending on the spices you use. The base is made ahead of time and stored in a glass jar. When you'd like some tea, add 1/2 to 1 teaspoon of the Turmeric Paste to a cup of warmed coconut, almond or raw milk.

bit.ly/GoldenMILK

Turmeric Paste

6 T Turmeric

1 T Cardamom

1/2 tsp Coriander

1/4 tsp Ginger, powdered

1/8 tsp Clove, ground

1 T Cinnamon, ground

1 C Purified water

Combine all ingredients in saucepan. Heat until thickened. Cool and then spoon into glass jar with tight fitting lid. When preparing the tea, add 1/2 - 1 tsp of paste to warmed milk of your choice.

Overnight Oatmeal

Traditional boxed cereals are processed and usually loaded with extra sugars. When grains are soaked overnight, the natural enzymes are activated to assist in the digestion of the grain. Ancient cultures made it a traditional practice to soak grains overnight in water to begin this process. Adding a protein to your oatmeal like nuts or seeds will form a complete protein that enhances the nutrient absorption and provides longer lasting sustenance. This overnight oatmeal makes a hearty breakfast and energizing start to your day. Some recipes call for soaking oats in dairy-free milk like coconut. If you'd like, soak them in purified water for the same result. Mix up the add-ins to meet your tastes. Keep in mind that chia seeds are a thickener. If you add them to your oats soak, add an extra spoonful of water for every spoonful of chia seed you mix in.

http://bit.ly/overnightOATMEAL

1/4 C Rolled Oats (if you have a wheat allergy, make sure they are "gluten free"

1/4 C Purified water or coconut milk/water

2-4 T fresh berries

Optional add-ins: 1 tsp pumpkin seeds, chia seeds, sesame seeds, almonds, walnuts or other nuts and seeds, pinch of cinnamon, nutmeg or cardamom

Pour oats in a ceramic or glass dish with a lid. Cover with purified water or coconut milk/water. Gently stir in berries keeping them whole or crushing them. Leave on the counter or in refrigerator 6-8 hours or overnight. In the morning, stir gently and enjoy for a satisfying breakfast! If you'd like them warm, gently heat in a stainless steel sauce pan just until warm. Do not overcook!

Fermented Veggies

Fermented vegetables are similar to Sauerkraut which is mainly made from cabbage. Fermenting veggies not only preserves them, but it produces healthy bacteria for your gut that supports proper digestion of proteins and carbohydrates. You can use a fermentation starter or the brine solution in this recipe. If your veggies become soggy, soft or develop an unpleasant odor, or mold grows in the solution toss them out.

bit.ly/FermentedVEGGIES

1 glass quart jar

1 1/2 T Celtic sea salt

2 C filtered water

Your choice of chopped veggies: Beets, broccoli, carrots, cauliflower, cabbage, kale, green beans, onions, herbs and spices.

1. Sterilize your glass jar by soaking in boiling water for 10 minutes. Remove and dry thoroughly.

2. Dissolve salt in water to make a Salt Brine.
3. Layer vegetables and spices in glass jar.
4. Leave 1-inch space at top of jar.
5. Cover veggies completely with Salt Brine.
6. Fold small cabbage leaf and press on veggies to submerge them in Brine.
7. Screw cap on tightly. (It's best to use a plastic cap rather than the metal caps which will oxidize and rust over time from the Brine solution.
8. Sit container on counter out of sunlight.
9. After 2-3 days, "burp" bottles 1-2 times a day.
10. Veggies should be soured in 5-8 days, sooner in warmer weather.
11. Move to the refrigerator for storage up to 3 months.

Carrot & Walnut Salad

(You can substitute any veggies of your choice)

Raw vegetables are very cleansing to our digestive system. If you are overcoming a stomach bug, it's more gentle to eat lightly cooked vegetables. Save the raw foods for when your digestive tract is needing some extra fiber to move things along. This basic vegetable salad makes a clean lunch option or side dish with a grilled meat and can be used with many vegetables, raw or lightly steamed. Beets, bok choy, broccoli, brussel sprouts, carrots, cauliflower, celery, kohlrabi, peppers, radishes.

bit.ly/RawCarrotBeetSalad

1/2 C Julienned carrots (cut into thin strips)

1/2 C Julienned beets

2 T Fresh parsley, chopped

1/4 C Chopped walnuts

Dressing

Carrot & Walnut Salad

2 T Olive oil

2 T Apple Cider Vinegar

1 T Organic sugar or Coconut Sap Sugar

Toss together cut vegetables and parsley. Mix together dressing ingredients and stir into vegetables, mix in walnuts and stir gently until combined.

Roasted/Grilled Veggies

2 C chopped vegetables

Simple combinations:

Bell peppers, red onion, tomatoes: toss in black olives and fresh basil after roasting.

Zucchini, eggplant, Vidalia onion, mushrooms: toss in fresh basil or oregano after roasting.

Sweet potato, green beans, yellow onions: toss in sliced almonds after roasting.

Preheat oven to 425 degrees Fahrenheit or put on "Broil". Line a cookie sheet with parchment paper. Chop up veggies of choice and place on the cookie sheet, drizzle with 1-2 tablespoons of Extra Virgin Olive Oil. Broil 5-10 minutes or until vegetables are gently cooked.

bit.ly/roastedVEGGIES

Basic Vinaigrette

Salad dressings are some of the easiest condiments to make and one of the most natural. Traditional salad dressings have preservatives, chemical flavorings like MSG (monosodium glutamate) and added sodium. Sidebar: Most packaged salad dressings are now made with soybean oil, one of the most genetically modified crops to withstand Round up weed killer.

These salad dressings can be mixed up as single use or multiplied in quantity for family size. Use glass jelly jars with a screw on lid to make it easy to shake before use.

Here are some simple salad dressing you can make and adjust to suit your tastes. Mix all the ingredients together in a glass jar, shake well before pouring over salad greens or veggies. Multiply the ingredients to make a larger batch for your family or company.

Single Serving Italian Dressing

1 tsp apple cider vinegar

1 T Extra virgin olive oil

Pinch of Italian herbs

1 tsp Fresh shredded parmesan or Romano cheese

Fresh ground sea salt & pepper to taste

Single Serving Honey Dijon

1 tsp Balsamic vinegar

4 tsp Olive oil

1 tsp Stoneground mustard

Pinch of garlic salt or 1/2 clove of crushed garlic

Fresh ground sea salt & pepper to taste

Single Serving Asian Dressing

1 tsp Rice vinegar

1 T Sesame oil

1/2 Clove of crushed garlic

Pinch of ground ginger or 1/4 tsp fresh grated ginger root

1 tsp toasted sesame seeds

4-6 fresh cilantro leaves minced

Fresh ground sea salt & pepper to taste

Grilled Tarragon Chicken

3 pounds Boneless, skinless chicken breasts

Makes 12-14 servings

http://bit.ly/GrilledCHICKEN

Marinade

1 C Extra virgin olive oil (also called EVO)

1/4 C Rice vinegar

1/4 C Dijon mustard

2 T Fresh tarragon, minced

2 Cloves garlic, minced

Mix all ingredients in a blender until combined. Pour over chicken breasts in a ceramic or glass dish, cover and refrigerate for 4-6 hours or overnight for more flavor. Cook over a hot grill until done. Put cooked chicken into covered casserole dish immediately after cooking to seal in moisture. Serve on a bed of greens with fresh vegetables.

Slice up remaining chicken and use for meals the next couple of days or freeze for quick fast food when you need it.

Grilled chicken makes a great addition to:

- Sandwiches - Add sliced chicken breast to ciabatta roll with leaf lettuce, fresh avocado and tomato slice with a drizzle of olive oil.
- Quiche - Dice cooked chicken and toss into egg mixture for your quiche before cooking.
- Wraps - Layer sliced, cooked chicken, slice of havarti cheese, spinach leaves and bell pepper slices on a soft shell tortilla or large lettuce leaf, roll tightly and wrap in waxed paper for a satisfying lunch.
- Rice dishes - Add diced chicken to cooked rice along with some curried vegetables for an Indian flare.

Basic Meat Marinade

Alternate the vinegars, seasonings and add-ins. For example, make an Italian marinade with EVO, Apple Cider Vinegar, crushed garlic, basil and oregano. Often the dressing recipes can double as a marinade.

Pad Thai Noodles

These are our favorite for a quick to fix lunch on a cooler day. They're made with Asian-style rice noodles that are long and flat. Substitute 2 cups of shredded red and green cabbage for the noodles if you'd like a Grain-free alternative.

http://bit.ly/SimplePadThai

6 ounces Asian-style Rice Noodles

2-4 quart saucepan

Sauce

4 tsp Honey or Agave nectar

1 tsp Chili sauce (optional)

3 T Natural Peanut butter

2 tsp Rice Vinegar

Juice of 1 Lime

Add-Ins

2 Carrots, grated or julienned

1/4 C Cilantro, chopped

3 Green onions, sliced

1 C cooked Chicken breast, diced (optional)

Chopped peanuts for garnish (optional)

Heat water for cooking rice noodles. When the water comes to a boil, drop the noodles in and stir as they begin to soften. While they continue cooking, mix together ingredients for the sauce. Drain the noodles in a colander once they become tender. Stir in the vegetables and chicken, finishing with the sauce to coat all ingredients. Serve with some more cilantro and chopped nuts to garnish.

Coconut Flour Brownies

---

5 T organic cocoa powder

3/4 C butter

1 C sugar (I use Rapadura or Coconut Sap)

1 tsp vanilla

6 beaten eggs

3/4 C sifted coconut flour

1/2 tsp baking powder

1/2 tsp salt

optional add ins: 2-3 drops Food Grade, Therapeutic essential oils of choice: orange, peppermint, or cinnamon

1 C chopped walnuts or pecans

http://bit.ly/PaleoBROWNIES

In a saucepan heat chocolate and butter over low heat, stirring occasionally, until melted.

Remove from heat and mix in sugar, eggs and vanilla.

Stir in remaining ingredients.

Spread in a greased 8x8-inch pan for thick brownies, 9x13-inch pan for thinner brownies.

Make sure not to Over-Cook or they will be dry!

Bake at 350 degrees F (175 C) for 30 minutes. .

Cool slightly before cutting.

Chia Seed Pudding

1 C Nut milk, rice milk or hemp milk

1/4 C Chia seeds

Mix together milk and chia seeds. Shake or stir gently. Pour into 4 serving dishes. Refrigerate 2-3 hours or overnight. Serve with fresh fruit, nuts or preserves.

No-Bake Grain-free Protein Truffles & Paleo Granola

1/2 C Hemp seeds

1 C Dates

1/4 C Seeds, your choice: sesame seeds, pumpkin seeds, sunflower seeds

1/2 C walnuts, chopped fine

1/2 C almonds, chopped fine

1/4 C Brazil nuts, chopped fine

1/2 tsp Real Vanilla extract

Optional: Dark Chocolate

Blend all ingredients well and form into balls. Refrigerate. Optionally, dip truffles into dark chocolate and store in the refrigerator.

http://bit.ly/PaleoTruffles

For Grain Free Granola, skip the dates and vanilla. Chop up all nuts and seeds to a medium texture (don't pulverize them). Part of the appeal of the grain-free granola is to preserve some of the varied colors and textures. Sprinkle over a cup of yogurt or enjoy a few tablespoons with 1/4 cup of almond or coconut milk.

Almond Flour Muffins

2 C almond flour

2 tsp baking powder

1/4 tsp salt

1/2 C coconut oil, melted

1/3 C water (omit this if using fresh fruit like chopped apples)

3 T honey, coconut sap or rapadura sugar

4 eggs

1 tsp vanilla

Optional add-ins: chopped nuts, chopped dried fruit, chocolate chips, chopped apples, shredded cheese, herbs, bacon.

http://bit.ly/AlmondFlourMUFFINS

Apple cinnamon version: add 1/3 cup diced apple (to the liquid mixture), 2 tsp cinnamon, 1/4 tsp fresh ground nutmeg (to the dry ingredients) and omit the water.

- Preheat the oven to 350 degrees F.
- While the oven warms, melt the coconut oil in an oven proof dish while you mix together the other ingredients.
- Mix together dry ingredients: flour, salt, baking powder and sugar (if using honey, add to the liquid mixture).
- In another bowl, mix the liquid ingredients: coconut oil, eggs (adding the eggs one at a time, beating well after each one), water, honey, vanilla.
- Combine the dry and liquid ingredients, mixing well. (Don't worry about mixing too much, this recipe doesn't have gluten which makes tough muffins if overmixed)
- Spoon batter into greased or papercup lined muffin tins (I recommend using the papercup liners for this recipe)

Bake for 12-15 minutes

Remove from pan to cool on a wire rack, serve warm with fresh fruit or preserves.

Other hints: Rumford's baking powder is aluminum free. Yes, most other baking powders have aluminum in them! We make our own Baking Powder that is CORN-FREE, yes, most baking powders are made with corn starch.

Corn-Free, Gluten-Free Baking Powder

1/4 C Baking soda

2 T Arrowroot powder

1/2 C Cream of Tarter

Sift together all ingredients 3 times. Store in an air tight container.

Use in recipes as called for. Mixture may clump, sift before use if needed.

We use unbleached paper liners for my muffin cups. This recipes makes great mini-muffins: makes 24 mini's plus 4 full sized muffins. Enjoy!

No-Bake Pumpkin Seed Caramel Bars

Filling

1 cup raw, organic pumpkin seeds

1 ½ cups raw cashew or other nut flour (ground nuts)

½ cup raw, organic sunflower seeds (or seeds of your choice)

2/3 cup organic coconut flour

1 cup organic almond butter

Organic Caramel Sauce

¼ cup organic butter

1 ½ cups organic coconut palm sugar

1 generous tbsp organic coconut cream

1 tsp organic vanilla extract

Pinch of sea salt

Optional: 1-2 drops of cinnamon bark, clove or orange essential oil (just choose 1!)

1 tbsp organic coconut palm sugar

http://bit.ly/PumpkinSeedBars

Mix all filling ingredients and 1 C of the Caramel Sauce. Save the rest of the caramel sauce for apple or fruit dip another time. Press into a 9x13-inch pan and divide into bars after cooled. You can put them in the fridge for 15 -20 minutes to help them firm up. If desired, freeze separately for on the go snacks. I made some extra caramel sauce for garnish and sprinkled each serving with raw cocoa nibs. Enjoy!

Makes 3 dozen small bars

15 Food Staples For Natural Cooking

Aside from your fresh vegetables, fruits and grass-fed meats, these staples will help you be prepared to make a variety of meals.

1. **Natural oils:** Coconut, Olive, Sesame, Real Butter

2. **Gluten-Free Flours:** Almond, Rice, GF Mixes

3. **Dairy-Free Milk Alternatives:** Almond, Coconut, Rice, Hemp

4. **Whole Spices:** Celtic sea salt, cinnamon, garlic, ginger, peppercorns, turmeric

5. **Raw Honey:** Local if you can find it

6. **Baking Soda & Baking Powder:** Aluminum and corn free

7. **Natural Vinegars:** Apple Cider (ACV), Balsamic, Rice

8. **Herbal Teas:** Chamomile, Hibiscus, Peppermint, Turmeric

9. **Purified Water:** Reverse Osmosis Filter or those with added minerals

10. **Nuts:** Almonds, Brazil, Macadamia, Pistachios, Walnuts. Store in the refrigerator to maintain freshness

11. **Seeds:** Alfalfa, Chia, Hemp, Pumpkin, Sesame, Sunflower

12. **Dried Fruits:** Apricots, Blueberries, Cherries, Currants, Dates, Mango, Mulberries, Wolfberries. Choose ones that have no added sugar or preservatives or sulphates

13. **Whole Grains:** Variety of rices (Basmati, Jasmine, Wild), Quinoa, Gluten-free Oats

14. **Fresh Citrus Fruits:** Grapefruit, Lemon, Lime

15. **Beans & Legumes:** Black, Garbanzo, Great Northern, Kidney, Lentils, Navy, Split Pea

Two Inches of Wool

15 Beauty Foods

1. Almonds

2. Apple Cider Vinegar

3. Avocado

4. Blueberries

5. Cherries

6. Chia Seeds

7. Coconut

8. Dark Chocolate

9. Eggs

10. Fermented Foods: Kimchi, Kombucha, Sauerkraut

11. Herbs & Spices: Cinnamon, Garlic, Ginger, Turmeric

12. Pumpkin Seeds

13. Sprouts

14. Walnuts

15. Wolfberries

Two Inches of Wool

15 Foods To Support Healthy Liver & Kidneys

To nourish the body, eat them raw (except the Legumes & Potatoes) or juice them.

Liver	Kidneys
Aloe Vera	Asparagus
Bananas	Celery
Beets	Cranberries
Cucumber	Cucumber
Ginger	Parsley
Legumes (Kidney Beans)	Potatoes
Lemon	Pumpkin Seeds
Parsley	Watermelon

15 Hidden Sources of Corn

Non-Organic Corn crops in the USA are often GMO "Round-up Ready Corn" which allows the crop to be sprayed with Round Up Weed Killer, all the weeds die, but the GMO plant survives along with any pesticide residue. The finished corn product makes it into our consumer goods along with ready to eat produce. GMO corn products have been found in research to stress the kidneys. Avoid corn if you have any kidney weakness.

1. **Ice Cream & Frozen Yogurt** Most made with corn syrup rather than milk or cream.

2. **Gluten Free Baked goods and GF flour** Corn flour or corn starch is common substitute for wheat flours.

3. **Gluten Free Cereals and Baby Food**

4. **Condiments** Ketchup, barbecue sauce, salad dressings Corn syrup.

5. **Baking Powder** Made with corn starch and Baking Soda. DIY: 2 T Baking Soda + 4 T sifted together 2-3 times. Store in airtight container. Use equal measure.

6. **Vanilla extract and other flavorings** Thickened with Corn Syrup. DIY Vanilla extract with pure vanilla beans cut open, cover with high grade Vodka and let this rest 4-6 weeks to develop flavor. Use as you would in equal amounts as you would traditional extract for recipes.

7. **White Vinegar** Substitute Apple Cider Vinegar in recipes.

8. **Powdered Sugar** Corn starch fluffs up the sugar. Use organic powdered sugar without.

9. **Supplements** Specifically Vitamin C, E, and Ascorbic Acid.

10. **Iodized Salt** Added corn starch keeps granules from sticking together.

11. **Corn Syrup** Cheap sweetener and thickener in many processed foods and coffee drinks.

12. **Dextrin, Dextrose** Inexpensive sweeteners used in place of regular sugar.

13. **Caramel Flavoring & Coloring** Corn syrup sweetens to thicken flavorings and coffee syrups.

14. **Xanthan Gum** Thickener used in Gluten Free baked goods '

15. **Maltodextrin** Flavoring formed from corn, found in most processed foods including flavored potato chips, snacks and most gluten-free goods.

Spiroux de Vandomoir, Joel. et al. "A Comparison of the Effects of Three GM Corn Varieties on Mammalian Health." International Journal of Biological Sciences.2009; 5(7):706-726. doi:10.7150/ijbs.5.706

Two Inches of Wool

SPA RECIPES

Air Freshener
3-Ingredient Lotion
Tooth Polish
Bug Spray
Travel Oils
Foaming Soap
Calming Lavender Spray
Hand Cleaner
Joyful Body Spray
Lip Balm Freshener

Air freshener: bit.ly/airFreshener

3-ingredient Lotion bit.ly/diyLOTION

Tooth Polish bit.ly/toothPOLISH

Bug Spray bit.ly/bugSPRAY

Travel 1st Aid Oils bit.ly/TRAVELoils

Foaming Soap bit.ly/DIYfoamingSOAP

Calming Lavender Spray bit.ly/2Lavender

Hand Cleaner bit.ly/DIYhandCLEANER

Joyful Body Spray bit.ly/DIYbodySPRAY

Lip Balm bit.ly/glowingSkin

Extra for e-book

Body Butter bit.ly/diyLOTION

Body Scrub bit.ly/glowingSkin

Calming Roll-On bit.ly/MelissaEssentialOil

Cooling Foot Spray bit.ly/TRAVELoils

Air Freshener

Air Freshener

Traditional air fresheners are just a combination of man-made chemicals that are confusing our chemistry. They smell nice, but these chemicals have been connected to many side effects like headaches, mental fog, nausea, they've even been linked with hormone and thyroid disruption. Essential oils are the whole ingredient alternatives to these synthetic aromas. You can customize your spritzer to suit your personality and preferences and they'll support a healthy mind and body.

1 Eight ounce glass spray bottle

1 Drop unscented castille soap

10-20 drops essential oils of choice: YL Purification is cleansing and freshening

8 ounces purified water

Add 1 drop of castille soap to the glass bottle to emulsify the oil and water. Add in essential oils of choice, 10 drops for a gentle fragrance, up to 20 for a more purifying blend. Fill the remainder with the purified water and shake gently to mix before using.

3 Ingredient Lotion

3 Ingredient Lotion

The main purpose of lotions are to moisturize our skin, right? Traditional lotions carry preservatives, fillers and emulsifiers in addition to synthetic fragrance (labeled as "parfum" "perfume" or "fragrance") which is disrupting to our body's delicate chemistry. This lotion recipe is easy to make and a fun one to try out on your DIY journey.

Ingredients

1/4 C Vegetable Oil (Almond, Coconut, Jojoba, Sesame, NO soybean, canola or corn)

1/4 C Emulsifying Wax (Local beeswax or emulsifying beads from a specialty store)

1 1/4 C Hot purified water (Almost boiling)

Glass quart canning jar with lid

Instructions

1. Temper the glass canning jar by slowing warming it in a pan of hot water.

2. Remove with a hot pad and set on a hot pad to cool slightly while you mix the ingredients.

3. Melt vegetable oil and emulsifying wax in a small stainless steel sauce pan.

4. Pour in hot water CAREFULLY. **This step is critical in avoiding a mess!

5. Stir until fully incorporated, the consistency will be like milk.

6. Pour the lotion slowly into the glass canning jar making sure the jar is still slightly warm and put the cap on.

7. Gently shake the mixture every five minutes until the mixture sets.

8. Add 8-10 drops of essential oils of your choice in the middle of mixing ingredients.

Add 8-10 drops of essential oils when the lotion cools to customize to your needs:

Calming lotion: Roman chamomile, lavender & frankincense

Acne prone: Melaleuca alternifolia, Roman Chamomile

Eczema: Myrrh

Cooling Foot Lotion: Peppermint

Sunscreen: Add 1 T non-nano zinc oxide plus lavender to protect and support skin health (I ordered mine from WabiSabi baby.com)

Insect Repelling Lotion: Purifying blend, Peppermint, Cedarwood, Immune Immune Boosting Blend, Citronella (make sure it is not a chemical citronella oil, but pure plant extract). Add non-nano zinc oxide to make a bug repellent sunscreen

Tooth Polish

Tooth Polish

Traditional tooth pastes have controversial ingredients, preservatives and fillers that may be stressing our body's detox organs as well as sweeteners and artificial flavorings. Our mouth is one of the first places our body absorbs nutrients and chemicals as the mucous membranes and salivary glands absorb ingredients and quickly transport them throughout the body. This is a simple tooth polish that gets your teeth bright and clean. You can still make it without the vegetable glycerin which softens the mixture so it isn't so grainy, more a texture effect.

Ingredients

2 T Baking Soda

1 tsp Celtic Sea Salt

1 T Vegetable Glycerin (make sure you don't use glycerin from the drug store which is made from chemicals. Natural glycerin comes from plants and is considered a "food" product.

2-4 drops Essential Oils safe as Dietary Supplements: Peppermint, Spearmint, Clove, Tangerine, or Orange all support natural dental hygiene.

Instructions

1. Mix all ingredients in a glass jar with a lid. Keep a small plastic spatula with it so you can scoop out single servings and keep your polish fresh.

Bug Spray

Bug Spray

Essential oils are the life blood of plants. The oils protect the plants from pests and invasive plant species. These same oils can protect you from some pests that fly about during the warmer weather. If you are mixing up a spray for kids, skip the peppermint as it's too strong an oil for the littles.

Ingredients

15 Drops YL Purification essential oil blend

8 Drops Peppermint essential oil

8 Drops Lavender essential oil

8 Drops Cedarwood essential oil

1/4 tsp Neem oil

Purified water, aloe vera, witch hazel or apple cider vinegar to fill bottle

8 ounce Glass spray bottle

Instructions

1. Mix together essential oils with Neem oil in the glass bottle. Shake gently to mix all the oils. Add the filling liquid of your choice. Shake gently before using.

Travel Oils

Travel Oils

Pack these essential oils in an up cycled mint tin. Fill 1-2ml glass vials with each oil and label accordingly:

•*Lavender essential oil* - calms your nervous system down during travel and helps alleviate insomnia from jet lag. Lavender a gentle, calming oil that may support healthy skin and immune function. Combine a drop of lavender, lemon & peppermint and massage into lymph glands to cleanse system.

•*Lemon essential oil* - boosts the immune system and may energize you during travel. Lemon is also anti-bacterial, so drinking it in your water will give you added protection against local flora. A drop or two of lemon essential oil can help keep your hands clean when water isn't available.

•Immune Boosting Blend with Cinnamon/Clove/Rosemary/Lemon/Eucalyptus Radiata is your major defense against bacteria and viruses. Applying this immune boosting blend to the soles of your feet or abdomen to support immune system.

•***Peppermint essential oil*** is good for relieving muscle soreness from carrying heavy luggage. Breathe in from the bottle for an energy boost (without caffeine that will goof up your sleep cycles even more). Peppermint is also helpful for easing nausea from travel or illness. Sip a drop of peppermint essential oil in your glass water bottle to calm queasiness.

•***A Purifying Blend with lemongrass, citronella and melaleuca alternifolia*** is an excellent insect repellent. It also cleanses wounds and freshens the air to fight airborne bacteria. Rub it on your skin as a natural bug deterrent or on the soles of your feet to discourage spiders from invading your bedding. If you want to make your own air freshener for travel, you can spray your sheets with Purifying essential oils as extra protection against bed bugs.

Foaming Soap

Foaming Soap

Ready made soaps have thickeners, antibacterial agents and artificial colors and fragrance. The best hand cleaners are simple as the cleansing process is really the most important aspect of hand cleaning. Scrubbing hands thoroughly for 1-2 minutes and rinsing thoroughly will give you the most hygienic cleaning. This is a simple soap you can mix up quickly for any sink in your home.

Customize your soap blend to suit your mood or the season:

Citrus oils will brighten your mood and add a fresh aroma Cinnamon, Clove, Rosemary and Melaleuca are purifying when you need some extra cleansing in the bathroom or kitchen Lavender, Chamomile and Ylang Ylang will calm you down at the end of the day.

Ingredients

1 ounce Dr. Bronner's Baby Mild, unscented Castile soap

3 ounces purified water

Therapeutic Essential Oils

Foaming soap container

Instructions

1. Pour castille soap into container

2. Add 5-10 drops essential oils of your choice

3. Fill remainder with pure water, making sure not to fill past the foamer unit

Calming Lavender Spray

Calming Lavender Spray

Ingredients

10-15 drops Lavender Essential Oil

Purified water, or aloe vera to fill bottle (Here's where I get my aloe link to Vita-cost affiliate)

8 ounce Glass spray bottle

Instructions

1. Drop essential oils in the glass bottle. Shake gently before using.

2. Spritz skin to cool after sun exposure or spray your pillow at bedtime to calm down.

DIY Hand Cleaner

DIY Hand Cleaner

Skip the alcohol antibacterial cleaners when you make your own travel size hand cleaner to keep in your handbag or gym bag.

Ingredients

10-15 drops Essential Oils, Lavender, Tea Tree, Lemon, Palmarosa are good cleaners

Purified water, witch hazel or aloe vera to fill bottle

8 ounce Glass spray bottle or up cycled 15ml glass essential oil bottle

Instructions

1. Drop essential oils in the glass bottle. Add liquid and shake gently before using.

2. Apply a couple of drops or spray hands and rub palms together, air dry.

Joyful Body Spray

Joyful Body Spray

Trading out chemical perfumes for a natural essential oil blend will save you exposure to many hormone and thyroid disrupting chemicals. Essential oils smell more authentic too! Young Living's Joy blend is a beautiful, feminine combination that is soothing to the skin as well. Mix up this body spray and spritz on instead of synthetic body care products when you'd like to freshen up after the shower or spray on legs after shaving to hydrate skin.

Ingredients

10-15 drops Young Living's Joy Essential Oil

Purified water, or aloe vera to fill bottle

8 ounce Glass spray bottle

Instructions

1. Drop essential oils in the glass bottle. Shake gently before using.

2. Spritz skin to cool after sun exposure or spray your pillow at bedtime to calm down.

Simple Lip Balm

Simple Lip Balm

1 T Coconut oil, unrefined

2 Drops lavender essential oil (Dietary Supplement Grade)

1 Lip balm container

Warm coconut oil in a small pan on the stove over very low heat or in a small ceramic dish in the oven. Add essential oils and mix gently. Spoon carefully into a lip balm container. Store in the refrigerator.

Advanced Lip Balm - also makes a great cuticle moisturizer

Uses the "bain-marie" method (literally translates to water-bath)

1 Ounce Beeswax pellets

2 T Coconut oil

7 drops Jojoba oil

Vitamin E capsule

Essential Oils of choice: Lavender, Spearmint, Chamomile, Tangerine, Geranium

Place beeswax in ceramic dish with high sides into a pan with water. Only fill the water enough to boil and heat the beeswax to melt. Make sure the sides are high enough to prevent water from splashing into mixture. After the beeswax is melted, add in coconut, jojoba and Vitamin E oil. Turn off the heat and gently stir in 10 drops of essential oils of choice.

15 Natural Resources

For Cleaning & Personal Care

1. **Aloe Vera:** Gentle skin care. Ingredient for diluting essential oils.

2. **Baking soda:** Natural cleanser, deep cleaner when combined with vinegar.

3. **Castille Soap:** Pure soap with no added chemicals or fragrance. DIY hand soap.

4. **Celtic Sea Salt:** Natural body scrub, Deep cleansing bath.

5. **Essential Oil Diffuser:** Freshen and fragrance your home with natural plant extracts. Replaces synthetic room fresheners.

6. **Basic Set of Essential Oils:** Skin care, antioxidant support, home cleaning, air purifier. Cinnamon-clove Blend, Copaiba, Digestive Blend, Eucalyptus Blend, Helichrysum-Muscle Blend, Lavender, Lemon, Frankincense, Peppermint, Tea Tree.

7. **Empty Spray Bottles and glass containers:** For mixing up your own air fresheners, cleaning solutions, DIY personal care products.

8. **Facial Clays:** Deep skin cleaning with DIY masks. French Green, White, Rhassoul.

9. **Lemons:** Nutritional support, gentle cleansing of digestive tract, skin renewal.

10. **Magnesium Salts:** Muscle relaxant, use in a spa bath to hydrate and calm.

11. **Oxygen Bleach:** Natural whitening alternative to chlorine bleach.

12. **Upcycled T-shirts and towels** Natural cleaning rags, alternative to paper towel.

13. **Vegetable Glycerin:** Natural ingredient for DIY personal care recipes.

14. **Vegetable Oils:** Apricot, Coconut, Jojoba, Sesame for natural skin moisture.

15. **Vinegar:** Natural cleaner for countertops, bathrooms, floors. Chemical free laundry softener, natural hair rinse.

Two Inches of Wool

333

15 Supports for Sleep

1. **Engage in some gentle movement** a few hours before bed: mild exercise or simple stretches.

2. **Eat a lighter meal** earlier in the evening and avoid eating a heavy meal just before bedtime.

3. **Shut down the computer**, electronic devices and TV 1 hour before bed.

4. **Make your bedroom a sanctuary**: keep electronic devices out and charge them in another room. Keep clutter to a minimum to promote a sense of calm.

5. **Surround yourself with soothing colors**: blues and muted tones bring on the calm, bright colors stimulate our senses.

6. **Diffuse calming essential oils at bedtime**: frankincense (Boswellia carterii), cedarwood, copaiba, lavender, sandalwood, ylang ylang. Only use the highest quality oils as any fillers or additives may work against your efforts to relax or may bring on a chemical headache.

7. **Check prescription drug side effects** that may interrupt sleep patterns: drowsiness, insomnia, agitation, digestion affects can all impact your sleep quality.

8. **Drink a cup of calming tea**: chamomile, passion flower, valerian.

9. **Go to sleep at the same time each night**. Set your alarm to wake the same time each day even if your schedule is off.

10. **Use natural sleep aids like melatonin sparingly** as supplementing may interfere with your body's own production.

11. **Get your Vitamin D levels checked.** Low D levels will keep you wired at night.

12. **Eat calcium-magnesium rich foods** to calm down your system: almonds, blackstrap molasses, chia seeds, pumpkin seeds, walnuts, wolf berries.

13. **Eat foods high in tryptophan** which naturally triggers melatonin: nut butters and milks, turkey, bananas, dates, whole grain crackers.

14. **Avoid stimulating foods before bed**: alcohol, coffee, foods that stimulate the brain: chocolate, rich desserts, cheese, fermented veggies, bacon & ham, spinach, tomatoes.

15. **Keep your digestive tract and liver function running well.** (see Liver & Kidney health list) Back ups in your digestion may affect the quality of your sleep. If you are waking regularly around 3am, this may indicate toxicity of your liver.

Two Inches of Wool

15 Essential Oils

Body Systems They Support

Add 1-2 drops to a teaspoon of vegetable carrier oil: apricot, coconut, jojoba, or sesame and apply to areas as desired.

1. **Clove:** Immune System, Oral Hygiene, Home Cleaning.

2. **Copaiba:** Hair, Skin, Nails, Brain, Overall Wellness.

3. **Eucalyptus Radiata: Respiratory** & Sinus, Skin.

4. **Fennel:** Hormone Balance, Digestive Tract.

5. **Frankincense:** (Boswellia Carterii) Skin, Brain, Overall Wellness, Mood lifter.

6. **Geranium:** Skin, Hormone Balance, Immune Support.

7. **German Chamomile:** Skin, Digestive, Immune Support.

8. **Helichrysum:** Skin, Nerves, Liver.

9. **Lavender:** Skin, Brain.

10. **Lemon:** Brain, Liver, Home Cleaning.

11. **Melaleauca alternifolia:** (Tea Tree) Skin, Nails, Immune System, Home Cleaning.

12. **Palo Santo** Overall Wellness, Skin, Mood lifter.

13. **Peppermint:** Natural energy, Naturally cooling, Muscles & Joints.

14. **Rosemary:** Hair, Skin.

15. **Sandalwood:** Hair, Skin, Digestive.

Two Inches of Wool

15 Essential Oils For Liver and Kidney Health

Add 1-2 drops to a teaspoon of vegetable carrier oil: apricot, coconut, jojoba, or sesame and apply over liver or kidney area.

Liver

1. **Celery Seed**: Apium graveolens

2. **Cypress**: Cupressus sempervirens

3. **Geranium**: Pelargonium graveolens

4. **German Chamomile**: Matricaria recutita

5. **Helichrysum**: Helichrysum italics

6. **Ledum**: Ledum groenlandicum

7. **Lemon**: Citrus limon

Kidneys

8. **Clove**: Syzygium aromaticum

9. **Fennel**: Foeniculum vulgare

10. **Geranium**: Pelargonium graveolens

11. **Grapefruit**: Citrus paradisi

12. **Juiper**: Juniper osteosperma

13. **Lemon**: Citrus limon

14. **Roman Chamomile**: Chamaemelum nobile

15. **Sage**: Salvia officinalis

Most Common Mistakes of Essential Oil Users

1. Mixing oil and water Water and oil do not mix. In some situations a watery solution can assist the essential oil in dispersing, such as in a DIY toner recipe. If you get essential oils in your eyes, however, you wouldn't want to splash water on the eyes as this would make the oils spread further. Instead, use a vegetable carrier oil to dilute the EO.

2. Applying hot oils onto delicate skin Oils that are high in "phenols" are considered "HOT". They will not burn the skin with one application of a small area, but could be potentially irritating if used frequently or in high concentrations without diluting. Some oils in this category include: Basil, cassia, cinnamon, clove, oregano, tarragon, thyme, and winter savory. These oils should always be diluted when used.

3. Not repeating often enough Essential oils metabolize in the body in 60-90 minutes. If you are targeting specific health support, it is best to repeat an oil application every 60-90 minutes for several applications until the body is balanced. It is more effective to apply 1-2 drops at regular intervals than to apply a large amount 1 time.

4. Using too many oils all at once Essential oils are highly concentrated and only require 1-2 drops at a time to be used safely. Applying too many oils at one can place a burden on the body. This is especially true of adding EO's to bath water where water dispersal magnifies the absorption of oils faster than any other application and ingestion where the liver must process the concentrated plant oils. Usually, 2-4 drops of essential oil total is enough for a bath use, the exception being a blend that might be recommended by an aromatherapist.

5. Using powerful oils every day Essential oils are potent and concentrated. There are many essential oils that are excellent for personal care products and natural fragrance. Save the powerful essential oils for immune support when you need them, rather than using them as a "vitamin" and taken everyday. Repeated daily use of powerful immune blends allows your body to become comfortable with the supplement and may not respond as favorably when it needs an extra boost. Some stronger oils such as oregano may also affect gut flora so it is prudent to limit internal use for specific needs.oils. Usually, 2-4 drops of essential oil total is enough for a bath. It is safer to apply 2 drops to the body each hour for 5 hours than to apply 10 drops all at once and not repeat application.

Two Inches of Wool

Most Common Mistakes (cont)

6. Applying photo toxic oils onto skin before sun exposure Citrus oils in particular increase the body's sensitivity to sun. Because of this, you should avoid the application of these oils to sun exposed skin at least 12 hours before any sun exposure to avoid a sunburn.

7. Subjecting oil bottles to sunlight, heat and oxygen will diminish the quality of the oil, affecting it's therapeutic benefits. Always store essential oils in a cool, dry location - even the refrigerator - to maintain the best quality. If you carry EO's in your purse or handbag in the summer, keep an ice pack with them to keep them cool.

8. Mixing essential oils with man-made chemicals Essential oils are absorbed into the body very quickly. They penetrate the surface of the skin and enter the bloodstream within minutes. Because of this, you should not combine essential oils with any synthetic body care products since the essential oils will allow the man-made chemicals to enter the skin as well where you most likely do want this to happen. Use only the best ingredients you can with your pure essential oils. It's similar to cooking. If you created an organic salad with fresh vegetables you wouldn't top it with fruit loops or gatorade, right?

9. Using inferior oils for therapeutic use Since there are few regulations in the essential oil industry, manufacturers could put synthetic fragrance chemicals in their products and call them "essential oils". Because of this it's most important that you invest in essential oils of the highest quality where there is no doubt about purity or potency. Price is often an indicator, if a price seems too good to be true it is probably a product with chemical fillers and not worth purchasing. If an essential oil has any fillers in it, this lessens any therapeutic benefit and the added chemicals may actually be harmful. The best essential oils come from a company that grows the plants, harvests them, distills plant material on location and tests all oils for purity, potency and chemistry standards for a product worthy of your investment.

10. Touching the bottle orifice (the plastic insert that drops oils out) with your finger tip. Your skin's chemicals will contaminate the essential oils in your bottles if you touch the top. A better way to get a drop of essential oil is to tip the bottle slightly (not upside down or gravity may pull out several drops quickly, probably much more than you wanted) and wait for a drop to fall out into your palm or a mixing dish.

11. Assuming that a medical professional is knowledgeable with administering essential oils. Ask smart questions of any practitioner: How long have you personally been using oils? How long with patients? What is your training?

Two Inches of Wool

Resources

Personal care
Vitacost
Feminine Care products
Aubrey Aloe Vera
www.Vitacost.com

Ancient Minerals
Topical Calcium Magnesium Spray
Magnesium Salt bath minerals
www.ancient-minerals.com

Mountain Rose Herbs
Spices natural resources
Skin and body care
www.mountainRoseHerbs.com

Non-Toxic Living
EWG Environmental Working Group
Check out safety of consumer goods
www.EWG.org

EcoLunchboxes
Stainless Steel Bento Boxes
www.EcoLunchBoxes.com

CAUSEGEAR
Ethical Totes, Backpacks, Accessories
Made By Free Women
www.CAUSEGEAR.com

Mighty Nest
Non-Toxic Home products
Foods
bit.ly/Mighty-Fix

Blue Canoe
Organic cotton Clothing
www.BlueCanoe.com

Holy Yoga
www.HolyYoga.net

Yoga supply
Manduka
www.Manduka.com

Young Living
www.YoungLiving.com

Nuts, Seeds, Organic Foods
Wilderness Family Naturals
www.WildernessFamilyNaturals.com

Celtic Sea Salt
www.CelticSeaSalt.com

Natural Living Foods & Body Care
THRIVE
http://bit.ly/iTHRIVE

Tea
Rishi Teas
www.Rishi-Tea.com

Spiritual
Proverbs 31 Ministries
www.Proverbs31.org

Trafficking Survivor Resources
Lacey's Hope Project
www.LaceysHopeProject.org

Rebecca Bender Initiatives
www.RebeccaBender.org

Treasures L.A.
www.IamATreasure.com

Intervention
Alcoholics Anonymous
www.aa.org

Domestic Abuse Hotline
www.theHotline.org
1-800-799-SAFE (7233)

NAMI - National Mental Health Illness
www.NAMI.org

Polaris National Human Trafficking Hotline
1-888-373-7888

Soul-Nurturing Scriptures

God has created us to be fully alive in Mind-Body-Spirit and to love him with all our heart, soul, mind and strength. Invite God into every aspect of your life, He wants to be there! Write down your favorite bible verses that will keep your focus on our loving creator and put them in a place where you'll see them often. Stick it to a bathroom mirror, on the dashboard of your car. He is your strength, be reminded of that all throughout your day! Trust Him for wisdom and your plans will succeed.

"Rejoice always, pray continually, give thanks in all circumstances; for this is God's will for you in Christ Jesus." 1 Thessalonians 5:16-18

"If any of you lacks wisdom, he should ask God, who give generously to all without finding fault, and it will be given to him. But when he asks, he must believe and not doubt." James 1:5-6

"As the body without faith is dead, so faith without deeds is dead" James 2:26

"Extend forgiveness to keep your soul healthy: "Be kind and compassionate to one another, forgiving each other, just as Christ Jesus forgave you" Ephesians 4:32

"Everything is permissible for me, but not everything is beneficial" 1 Corinthians 6:12

"Search me, O God, and know my heart; test me and know my anxious thoughts. See if there is any offensive way in me and lead me in the way of everlasting." Psalm 139:23-24

Psalm 119 is 176 verses long. Much of it is about meditating on God's word, His laws, His wonders, His decrees, His statutes, His promises. Looking to God for understanding which is rooted in His word. Read through Psalm 119 and journal about which scriptures speak to you.

"Serve one another in love. Galatians 5:13

"My grace is sufficient for you, for my power is made perfect in weakness. Therefore, I will boast all the more gladly about my weakness's so that Christ's power may rest on me" 2 Corinthians 12:9-10

"My message and my preaching were not wise and persuasive words, but with a demonstration of the Spirit's power, so that your faith might not rest on men's wisdom, but on God's power." 1 Corinthians 2:4-5

"Do not conform any longer to the pattern of this world, but be transformed by the renewing of your mind. then you will be able to test and approve what God's will is-his good, pleasing and perfect will." Romans 12:1

"However, I consider my life worth nothing to me, if only I may finish the race and complete the task the Lord has given me-the task of testifying to the gospel of God's grace." Acts 20:24

"By wisdom a house is built, and through understanding it is established; through knowledge it's rooms are filled with rare and beautiful treasures." Proverbs 24:3-7

Bibliography

Balch, Phyllis, James Balch. Prescription for Nutritional Healing. Penguin Books. New York, New York. 2000.

Barnes, J., ed. *The Complete Works of Aristotle*, Volumes I and II, Princeton: Princeton University Press, 1984.

The Quest Study Bible, New International Version. Zondervan Publishing House. Grand Rapids, Michigan.

Bishop, Bryan. Boundless. Baker Books. Grand Rapids, Michigan. 2015.

Brown, Brene. Daring Greatly. Gotham Books. New York, New York. 2012

Blank, Martin. Overpowered, What Science Tells Us About the Dangers of Cell Phones and Other WiFi-Age Devices. Seven Stories Press. New York, New York. 2014.

Boon, Brooke. Holy Yoga. Faith Words. New York, New York. 2007.

Borba, Michele. UnSelfie, Why Empathetic Kids Succeed in Our

All-About-Me World. Touchstone Books. New York, New York. 2016.

Brown, Brene. Daring Greatly. Gotham Books. New York, New York. 2012.

Buckle, Jane. Clinical Aromatherapy. Elsevier. St. Louis, Missouri. 2015. 173-181.

Corbett, Steve, and Brian Fikkert. When Helping Hurts. Moody Publishers. Chicago, Illinois. 2012.

David, Dr. William. Wheat Belly. Rodale Books. Reprint edition June 2014.

DeMille, Oliver. "The Future of American Education". TJEd Online

Elderidge, John. The Journey of Desire. John Elderidge 2000.

Elderidge, John. Wild at Heart. Nelson Books. Nashville, Tennessee. 2001.

Elliot, Elisabeth. Discipline The Glad Surrender. Revell. Grand Rapids, Michigan. 1982.

Emerson, David. Overcoming Trauma through Yoga. North Atlantic Books. Berkeley, California. 2011.

Frawley, D. Yoga & Ayurveda. Lotus Press. 1999.

Gaarder, Jostein. Sophie's World, A Novel About The History Of Philosophy. Farrar, Straus, and Giroux. New York, New York. 1994.

Giglio, Louie. Wired For a Life of Worship. Multnomah Publishers. 2006.

Greitens, Eric. Resilience. Mariner Books. New York, New York. 2015.

Gresh, Dannah. Get Lost. Waterbrook Press. Colorado Springs, Colorado. 2001.

Gross P, Zhang R, Zhang X. "Wolfberry, Nature's Bounty of Nutrition and Health." BookSurge, LLC. 2006.

Henle, Mary. Documents of Gestalt Psychology: Solomon Asch, "Effects of Group Pressure Upon The Modification and Distortion of Judgements." Swathmore College. University of California Press. Berkely, California. 1961.

Houston, Brian. Live, Love, Lead. FaithWords. New York, New York. 2015.

Hybels, Bill. Simplify. Tyndale House Publishers, Inc. Carol Stream, Illinois. 2014.

Katzen, Mollie. Moosewood Cookbook. Ten Speed Press. Kensington, California. 1997.

Kersting, Thomas. Disconnected. How To Reconnect Our Digitally Distracted Kids. Thomas Kersting. United States. 2016.

King James Bible. Holman Bible Publishers. Nashville, Tennessee. 1979.

Leaf, Caroline. Switch on Your Brain. Baker Books. Grand Rapids, Michigan. 2013.

Ley, Emily. Grace Not Perfection. Thomas Nelson. Nashville, Tennessee. 2016

Long, Ray. The Key Poses of Yoga. Volume 1. Raymond A. Long. China. 2005.

Margoles, Michael. Chronic Pain. Taylor and Francis. 1998.

Maxwell, John. Intentional Living. Hachette Book Group. New York, New York. 2015.

McNeal, Reggie. A Work of Heart. Jossey-Bass. San Francisco, California. 2011.

Mother Teresa. No Greater Love. New World Library. Novato, California. 1989.

Niequist, Shauna. Savor. Zondervan. Grand Rapids, Michigan. 2015.

Ober, Clinton, Stephen T Sinatra, Martin Zucker. Earthing. Basic Health Publications. Laguna Beach, California. 2014.

Ortberg, John. Soul Keeping. Zondervan. Grand Rapids, Michigan. 2014.

Osteen, Joel. The Power of I Am. Hachette Book Group. New York, New York. 2015.

O'Donohue, John. Anam Cara, A Book of Celtic Wisdom. Harper Collins Publishers, Inc. New York, New York. 1997.

Richardson, Lisa Boalt. Modern Tea. Chronicle Books. San Francisco, California. 2014.

Ross, Julia. The Mood Cure. Viking Penguin Group. New York, New York. 2000.

Strong, James. Strong's Exhaustive Concordance of the Bible. Thomas Nelson Publishers. 1990.

Schwartz G, "In Bad Taste: The M.S.G. Syndrome. Signet Publishing. New York, New York. 1988.

Stanford Encyclopedia of Philosophy. 2008.

Terkeurst, Lysa. The Best Yes. Nelson Books. Austin, Texas. 2014.

Thomas, Gary. Sacred Pathways. Zondervan. Grand Rapids, Michigan. 2010. 50.

Valnet, Jean. The Practice of Aromatherapy. Healing Arts Press. Rochester, Vermont. 1990. 49.

Van Der Kolk, Bessel. *The Body Keeps The Score, Brain, Mind and Body in the Healing of Trauma.* New York: Penguin Books, 2014.

Warren, Rick. The Purpose Driven Life. Zondervan. Grand Rapids, Michigan. 2002.

Webster's Elementary Dictionary. G. & C. Merriam Co. 1941.

Whyte, David. The Heart Aroused. Currency Paperback. New York, New York. 1994.

Woodward, Orrin. Resolved. Obstacles Press. Inc. Flint, Michigan. 2011.

Worwood, Valerie Ann. The Complete Book of Essential Oils & Aromatherapy. New World Library. San Rafael, California. 1991.

Aaron, Ruth. Super Baby Food. F.J. Roberts Publishing Company. Peckville, Pennsylvania.

Zacharias, Ravi. Jesus Among Other Gods. Thomas Nelson. Nashville, Tennessee. 2000.

Zand, Janet, Rachel Walton, Bob Rountree. Smart Medicine for a Healthier Child. Avery Publishing Group. Garden City Park, New York. 1994.

Endnotes

1. O'Donohue, John. Anam Cara, A Book of Celtic Wisdom. Harper Collins Publishers, Inc. New York, New York. 1997. 135.

2. Gresh, Dannah. Get Lost. Waterbrook Press. Colorado Springs, Colorado. 2001. 86. Based on Psalm 51:7, Romans 4:17, Psalm 119:105, James 1:22, 2 Corinth 1:3-4.

3. DeMille, Oliver. "The Future of American Education". TJEd Online

4. Ortberg, John. Soul Keeping. Zondervan. Grand Rapids, Michigan. 2014. 43.

5. Strong, James. Strong's Exhaustive Concordance of the Bible. Thomas Nelson Publishers. 1990. Hebrew and Chaldee Dictionary. 114.

6. The Quest Study Bible, New International Version. Zondervan Publishing House. Grand Rapids, Michigan. 1644.

7. Peterson, Eugene. Eat This Book. William B Erdman Publishing. Colorado Springs, CO. 2006. 2

8. CDC. "9 Million Americans Use Sleeping Pills." NY Daily News. N.p., 30 Aug. 2013. Web. 27 July 2017.

9. Erdos, Joseph. "America's Coffee Obsession: Fun Facts That Prove We're Hooked." The Huffington Post. TheHuffingtonPost.com, 29 Sept. 2011. Web. 27 July 2017.

10. Duncan, Eric. "Topic: Energy Drinks." www.statista.com

11. www.statista.com Find statistics, consumer survey results and industry studies from over 18,000 sources on over 60,000 topics on the internet's leading statistics database.

12. "U.S.: Most Used Brands of Air Freshener Sprays and Room Deodorizers 2016 | Statistic." Statista. N.p., n.d. Web. 27 July 2017.

13. Greitens, Eric. Resilience. First Mariner Books. New York, New York. 2016. 108.

14. Ley, Emily. Grace Not Perfection. Thomas Nelson. Nashville, Tennessee. 2016. 186.

15. Van Der Kolk, Bessel. *The Body Keeps The Score, Brain, Mind and Body in the Healing of Trauma.* New York: Penguin Books, 2014. 281.

16. Maxwell, John. Intentional Living. Hachette Book Group. New York, New York. 2015. 14.

17. Mother Teresa. No Greater Love. New World Library. Novato, California. 1989. 25.

18. The Quest Study Bible, New International Version. Zondervan Publishing House. Grand Rapids, Michigan. 1341.

19. Ibid. 1348.

20. Ibid. 812.

21. Warren, Rick. The Purpose Driven Life. Zondervan. Grand Rapids, Michigan. 2002. 31.

22. Houston, Brian. Live, Love, Lead. FaithWords. New York, New You. 2015. 169.

23. Goetschel, Chuck. Simon Says. Obstacles Press, Inc. Grand Blane, Michigan. 2009.

24. Webster's Elementary Dictionary. G. & C. Merriam Co. 1941. 726.

25. McNeal, Reggie. A Work of Heart. Jossey-Bass. San Francisco, California. 2011. 41.

26. Zacharias, Ravi. Jesus Among Other Gods. Thomas Nelson. Nashville, Tennessee. 2000. 86.

27. The Message, The Bible In Contemporary Language. NavPress. Colorado Springs, Colorado. 2016.

28. Brown, Richard, Patricia Gerbarg. The Healing Power of the Breath. Shambhala. Boston, Massachusetts. 2012. 124.

29. O'Donohue, John. Anam Cara, A Book of Celtic Wisdom. Harper Collins Publishers, Inc. New York, New York. 1997. 106.

30. Aristotle. Stanford Encyclopedia of Philosophy. 2008. https://plato.stanford.edu/entries/aristotle/

31. Van Der Kolk, Bessel. *The Body Keeps The Score, Brain, Mind and Body in the Healing of Trauma.* New York: Penguin Books, 2014. 98.

32. "Violence in the Media, History of Research on." Encyclopedia of Communication and Information. Encyclopedia.com. 22 Aug. 2017 http://www.encyclopedia.com

33. Knowing Jesus. Sight In The Bible. https://bible.knowing-jesus.com/words/Sight

34. The Holy Bible, English Standard Version (ESV). Crossway. Wheaton, Illinois. 2001. 2.

35. Bible Gateway. Paul's Conversion. Acts 9 Commentary. https://www.biblegateway.com/resources/commentaries/IVP-NT/Acts/Pauls-Conversion.

36. The Holy Bible, English Standard Version (ESV). Crossway. Wheaton, Illinois. 2001. 396.

37. O'Donohue, John. Anam Cara, A Book of Celtic Wisdom. Harper Collins Publishers, Inc. New York, New York. 1997. 135.

38. Environmental Working Group, "Not so Sexy, Hidden chemicals in perfume and cologne." May 2010.

39. Elderidge, John. The Journey of Desire. Thomas Nelson Publishers. Nashville, Tennessee. 2000. 61.

40. Henle, Mary. Documents of Gestalt Psychology: Solomon Asch, "Effects of Group Pressure Upon The Modification and Distortion of Judgements." Swathmore College. University of California Press. Berkely, California. 1961. 221-235.

41. National Cancer Institute. "Cell Phones and Cancer Risk". June 2012.

42. Boon, Brooke. Holy Yoga. Faith Words. New York, New York. 2007.

43. James, Todd. Hatha Yoga Family Tree. Yoga Journal. 2001. 106-107.

44. King James Bible. Holman Bible Publishers. Nashville, Tennessee. Colossians 2:9. 685.

45. Ibid, 624.

46. Ibid.

47. Ibid, 621.

48. Ibid.

49. Ibid, 622.

50. Zacharias, Ravi. Jesus Among Other Gods. Thomas Nelson. Nashville, Tennessee. 2000. 89.

51. Ogden and K. Minton. "Sensorimotor Psychotherapy: One

Method for Processing Traumatic Memory." Traumatology 6, no. 3. 2000

52. Rhodes, Alison. "Claiming Peaceful Embodiment Through Yoga In The Aftermath Of Trauma". Complimentary Therapies In Clinical Practice. 21 (2015) 247-256.

53. Price, Maggi. et. al. "Effectiveness of an Extended Yoga Treatment For Women with Chronic Posttraumatic Stress Disorder". Journal of Alternative and Complimentary Medicine. Volume 23. Number 4. 2017. 300-309.

54. Rhodes, Alison. Joseph Spinazzola, Bessel van der Kolk. "Yoga For Adult Women With PTSD: A Long Term Follow-Up Study". Journal of Alternative And Complementary Medicine. Volume 22, Number 3. 2016. 189-196.

55. Vance, Heidi. Trauma Sensitive Holy Yoga Lecture. April 2017.

56. ENCODE Project. Press Release: ENCODE Data Describes Function Of Human Genome. Sept 5, 2012. http://bit.ly/ENCODEdata9_5_12

57. Silva, M, M Shyam, B.K.S. Iyengar. "Yoga the Iyengar Way." Dorling Kindersley. 1990.

58. The Bible, New International Version. Colorado Springs, Colorado. 1978. 1391.

59. Ibid. 858.

60. Porges, S.W. "The Polyvagal Theory: New Insights into Adaptive Reactions of the Autonomic Nervous System." Cleveland Clinic Journal of Medicine. 76, no. 2. (2009): S86-S90.

61. Encyclopedia of World Biography. The Gale Group Inc. 2004. Nebuchadnezzar.http://www.encyclopedia.com/people/history/ancient-history-middle-east-biographies/nebuchadnezzar

62. Grosso, Giuseppe, Fabio Galvano, Stefano Marventano, Michel Malaguarnera, Claudio Bucolo, Filippo Drago, Filippo Caraci.

Omega-3 Fatty Acids and Depression: Scientific Evidence and Biological Mechanisms. Oxidative Medicine and Cellular Longevity. Volume 2014 (2014), Article ID 313570. http://dx.doi.org/10.1155/2014/313570

63. Cook, J.D. E.R. Monsen. Vitamin C, The Common Cold, and Iron Absorption. The American Journal of Clinical Nutrition. February 1977. Vol. 30 no. 2 235-241.http://ajcn.nutrition.org/content/30/2/235.short

64. Rayne, Sierra. Concentrations and Profiles of Melatonin and Serotonin in Fruits and Vegetables During Ripending: A Mini-Review. Ecologica Research. British Columbia, Canada. http://bit.ly/2fI79q8

65. Margoles, Michael. Chronic Pain. Taylor and Francis. 1998.

66. Gross P, Zhang R, Zhang X. "Wolfberry, Nature's Bounty of Nutrition and Health." BookSurge, LLC. 2006. 25.

67. Held, K. et al. Oral Mg Supplementation Reverses Age-Related Neuroendocrine and Sleep EEG Changes In Humans. Pharma-copsychiatry. 2002; 35(4): 135-143. https://www.thieme-connect.de/DOI/DOI?10.1055/s-2002-33195#R127-59

68. Hudson, C.J. S.P. Hudson. Tryptophan Source From Plants And Uses Therof. US Patent 6,503,543. 2003.

69. Crinnion, Walter J. "Organic foods contain higher levels of certain nutrients, lower levels of pesticides, and may provide health benefits for the consumer." *Alternative Medicine Review*, Apr. 2010, p. 4+. *Academic OneFile.*

70. *Ghusoon, et. al. Assessment The Therapeutic Effects of Aqueous Extracts of Cilantro and Garlic In Mercuric Chloride Poisoning In Rats. The Iraqi J. Vet. Med. 2012; 36 (2):231-243.*

71. *California Department of Pesticide Regulation, Pesticide Residues on Fresh Produce. 2015. Available at* www.cdpr.ca.gov/docs/enforce/residue/resi2015/rsfr2015.htm.

72. *Trayyem RF, Health DD, Al-Delaimy WK, Rock CL. "Curcumin Content of Turmeric and Curry Powders." Nutr Cancer: 2006: 55(2); 126-131.*

73. *Schramm, Derek D, Malina Karim, Heather Schrader, Roberta Holt, Marcia Cardetti, Carl Keen. "Honey with High Levels of Antioxidants Can Provide Protection to Healthy Human Subjects." Journal of Agricultural Food and Chemistry. February 2003. 1732-1735.*

74. *Gross P, Zhang R, Zhang X. "Wolfberry, Nature's Bounty of Nutrition and Health." BookSurge, LLC. 2006.*

75. Dr. Mercola. Avoid Drinking Pasteurized Milk Until You Read These Details. April 2010. http://articles.mercola.com/sites/articles/archive/2010/04/27/do es-drinking-milk-cause-upperrespiratory-congestion.aspx

76. Kretowicz, Marek, Richard J. Johnson, Takuji Ishimoto, Takahiko Nakagawa, and Jacek Manitius. The Impact of Fructose on Renal Function and Blood Pressure. International Journal of Nephrology. Volume 2011 (2011), Article ID 315879, 5 pages http://dx.doi.org/10.4061/2011/315879

77. Grotheer, P, Marshall, M, Simonne, A. "Sulfites: Separating Fact from Fiction". University of Florida IFAS Extension. April 2005.

78. Rowe, KS, KJ Rowe. "Synthetic food coloring and behavior: A dose-response effect in a double-blind, placebo-controlled, repeated measures study." J Pediatr. 1994;125(5 Pt 1):691-98.

79. Schwartz G, "In Bad Taste: The M.S.G. Syndrome. Signet Publishing. New York, New York. 1988.

80. Flythe, Jennifer E., Jose F. Rueda, Michael K. Riscoe, Suzanne Watnick. "Silicate Nephrolithiasis After Ingestion of Supplements Containing Silica Dioxide." American Journal of Kidney Diseases Volume 54, Issue 1, July 2009, Pages 127–130. http://www.sciencedirect.com/science/article/pii/S027263860801 6132

81. Tobacman, J K. "Review of harmful gastrointestinal effects of

carrageenan in animal experiments." Environ Health Perspect. 2001 Oct; 109(10): 983–994. https://www.ncbi.nlm.nih.gov/pmc/articles/PMC1242073/

82. Thornton, J. "Is This the Most Dangerous Food For Men?". www.menshealth.com/nutrition/soys-negative-effects. May 2009.

83. Divi RL, Chang IIC, Doerge DR. "Anti-thyroid isoflavones from soybean: Isolation, characterization, and mechanisms of action." Biochem Pharmacy 1997. November 15;54(10):1087-96.

84. Nagata C, S. Inaba, N. Kawakami, T. Kakizoe, H. Shimizu. "Inverse association of soy product intake with serum adrogen and estrogen concentrations in Japanese men." Nutr Cancer. 2000;36(1):14-18.

85. White, LR, H Petrovich, GW Ross, KH Masaki. "Association of mid-life consumption of tofu with late life cognitive impairment and dementia: The Honolulu-Asia Aging Study." Fifth International Conference on Alzheimer's Disease. #487, 1996 July 27. Osaka, Japan.

86. Ross, Julia. The Mood Cure. Viking Penguin Group. New York, New York. 2000. 133.

87. Glover, James B., Marisa E. Domino, Kenneth C. Altman, James W. Dillman, William S. Castleberry, Jeannie P. Eidson, Micheal Mattocks. "Mercury in South Carolina Fishes USA." Ecotoxicology April 2010, Volume 19, Issue 4, pp 781–795.

88. www.nationalcandidacenter.com/candida-self-exams/.

89. Amen Clinics. Drinking Decreases Number of New Brain Cells. November 2012. http://www.amenclinics.com/blog/drinking-decreases-number-of-new-brain-cells/

90. Ballenger, James. Frederick Goodwin, Leslie Major. Alcohol and Central Serotonin Metabolism in Man. Arch Gen Psychiatry. 1979, 36(2):224-227.

91. Cell Press. Antibiotics That Kill Gut Bacteria Also Stop The

Growth Of Brain Cells. Science Daily. May 19, 2016. http://bit.ly/2vSilXZ

92. Klarer, Melanie, Myrtha Arnold, Lydia Günther, Christine Winter, Wolfgang Langhans and Urs Meyer. "Gut Vagal Afferents Differentially Modulate Innate Anxiety and Fear." Journal of Neuroscience 21 May 2014, 34 (21) 7067-7076; DOI: https://doi.org/10.1523/JNEUROSCI.0252-14.2014

93. McIntosh, James. Serotonin: Facts, What does Serotonin do? Medical News Today. Updated April 29, 2016. http://www.medicalnewstoday.com/kc/serotonin-facts-232248

94. Nahas Z , Marangell LB , Husain MM , Rush AJ , Sackeim HA , Lisanby SH , Martinez JM .Two-year outcome of Vagus Nerve stimulation (VNS) for treatment of depressive episodes. The Journal of Clinical Psychology/ 01 Sep 2005, 66(9):1097-1104.

95. Van Der Kolk, Bessel. The Body Keeps the Score. Penguin Books. New York, New York. 2014. 98.

96. National Institute of Health. NIH Human Microbiome Project Defines Normal Bacteria Makeup Of The Body. U.S. Department of Health & Human Services. News Release, June 2012. http://bit.ly/NIHstudyMicrobiome.

97. Bravo, et. al. Ingestion of Lactobacillus Strain Regulates Emotional Behavior and Central GABA Receptor Expression in a Mouse Via The Vagus Nerve. Proc. Natil. Acad Sci USA. 2011. Sept 20;108(38).https://www.ncbi.nlm.nih.gov/pubmed/21876150

98. Shaw G, et. al. "Stress Management for Irritable Bowel Syndrome: A Controlled Trial." Digestion 1991;50:36-42. https://doi.org/10.1159/000200738

99. Konturek, P.C. T. Brzozowski, S.J. Konturek. The Gut: Pathophysiology, Clinical Consequences, Diagnostic Approach And Treatment Options. Journal of Physiology and Pharmacology. 2001. 62.6. 591-599.

100. David, Dr. William. Wheat Belly. Rodale Books. Reprint edition June 2014.

101. Holmes, Kanina. "Monsanto Frantically Recalls GE Canola Seed in Canada." Organic Consumers Association. https://www.organicconsumers.org/old_articles/gefood/canolarecall.php

102. U.S. Canola Association. "What is Canola?" http://www.uscanola.com/what-is-canola/

103. Policiano, A. the Watermelon Cleanse. www.doctorariel.blogspot.com. August 2007.

104. Lozniewski, a, Haristoy, X, et al. "Dietary Component Kills Bacterial Cause of Ulcers and Stomach Cancers". John Hopkins Medicine. May 2002.

105. Lotito,S PhD. "Why Apples are Healthful." Linus Pauling Institute. November 2004.

106. Rivlin, Richard. "Historical Perspective on the Use of Garlic." The Journal of Nutrition. 2001.

107. Neil, Andrew, Christopher Silagy. "Garlic: It's Cardio-protective Properties." Lipidology. February 1994.

108. Fallon, S. Nourishing Traditions. New Trends Publishing. 1999.103.

109. Vicente Micol, Helen Larson, Bejit Edeas, Takuya Ikeda. Watermelon extract stimulates antioxidant enzymes and improves glycemic and lipid metabolism. Instituto de Biologia Molecular y Celular. http://www.teknoscienze.com/agro/pdf/micol-Ninapharm.pdf

110. Sawsan Ibrahim Kreydiyyeh, Julnar Usta. Diuretic effect and mechanism of action of parsley. Journal of Ethnopharmacology. Volume 79, Issue 3, March 2002. 353-357.

111. Pritchard, J. "Grapefruit and Kidney Stones." www.livestrong.com. June 2011.

112. Di Muro, Fabrizio, Kyle B. Murray. "An Arousal Regulation Explanation of Mood Effects on Consumer Choice." Journal of Consumer Research. Volume 39, Issue 3, 1 October 2012.

113. Warrenburg, Stephen. "Effects of Fragrance on Emotions: Mood and Physiology." Chem Senses (2005) 30 (suppl_1): i248-i249.

114. Cellier,D, Gilles-Eric,S, et al. "A Comparison of the Effects of Three GM Corn Varieties on Mammalian Health." Int J Biol Sci. 2009; 5(7):706-726. don;10.7150/rjbs.5.706.

115. Richardson, Lisa Boalt. Modern Tea. Chronicle Books. San Francisco, California. 2014. 146.

116. University of Maryland Medical Center. "Green Tea as an Antioxidant." October 2011. www.umm.edu/altmed/articles/green-tea-000255.htm.

117. Richardson, Lisa Boalt. Modern Tea. Chronicle Books. San Francisco, California. 2014. 77.

118. Natural Resources Defense Council. Clean by Design, Cotton Factsheet. August 2011.

119. Worwood, Valerie Ann. The Complete Book of Essential Oils & Aromatherapy. New World Library. San Rafael, California. 1991. 7.

120. Safe Handwashing. www.cdc.gov/Handwashing/

121. Komori, T, R. Fujiwara, M. Tanida, et al. "Effects of Citrus Fragrance on Immune Function and Depressive States." Neuroim-munodulation. 1995 (2): 174-180.

122. Valnet, Jean. The Practice of Aromatherapy. Healing Arts Press. Rochester, Vermont. 1990. 49.

123. Wang, Sam. The Neuroscience of Everyday Life. The Teaching Company. Chantilly, Virginia. 2010. 52.

124. Buckle, Jane. Clinical Aromatherapy. Elsevier. St. Louis, Missouri. 2015. 173-181.

125. Zand, Janet, Rachel Walton, Bob Rountree. Smart Medicine for a Healthier Child. Avery Publishing Group. Garden City Park, New York. 1994. 284.

126. Chen, Ying-Ju. "Inhalation of Neroli Essential Oil and It's Anxiolytic Effects." Journal of Complementary and Integrative Medicine. June 20, 2008. https://doi.org/10.2202/1553-3840.1143

127. Przybylski, Andrew, Netta Weinstein. "Can You Connect With Me Now? How the Presence of Mobile Communication Technology Influences Face-to-Face Conversation Quality." Journal of Social and Personal Relationships. 30, no 3. 2012. 237-46.

128. Kersting, Thomas. Disconnected. How To Reconnect Our Digitally Distracted Kids.Thomas Kersting. United States. 2016. 39.

129. Evangelista, Benny. "Attention Loss Feared as High-Tech Rewires Brain." San Francisco Chronicle. November 15, 2009.

130. Atasoy HI, MY Gunal, P Ataloy, S Elgun, G. Bugdayci. Immunohistopathologic demonstration of deleterious effects on growing rat testes of radio frequency waves emitted from conventional Wi-Fi devices. J Pediatric Urology. March 2012.

131. De Iuliis, GN, RJ Newey, BV King, RJ Aitken. "Mobile Phone Radiation Induces Reactive Oxygen Species Production and DNA Damage in Human Spermatozoa In Vitro. Pos ONE 4(7): e6446. doi:10.1371/journal.pone.0006446.

132. Balci, M, E Devrim, I Durak. "Effects of mobile phones on oxidant/antioxidant balance in the cornea and lens of rats. Curr Eye Res. 32(1):21-25, 2007.

133. Burch, J.B., "Melatonin Metabolite Excretion Among Cellular Telephone Users." International Journal of Radiation Biology 78, no 11. (2002): 1029-1036.

134. Salford, Leif, et. al. "Permeability of the Blood-Brain

Barrier Induced by 915 MHz Electromagnetic Radiation, Continuous Wave and Modulated at 8, 16, 50, and 200 Hz." Microscopy Research and Technique 27, no. 6. (1994); 535-542.

135. Frey, Allan H. "Human Auditory System Response to Modulated Electromagnetic Energy." Journal of Applied Psychology 17, no. 4 (1962). 689-692.

136. Andrew A. Marino, Erik Nilsen, Clifton Frilot, Nonlinear Changes in Brain Electrical Activity Due to Cell Phone Radiation. Bioelectromagnetics 24:339 346 (2003)

137. Baldwin, Roberto. "Keep Your Computer From Destroying Your Eyesight." Gear. September 5, 2013. https://www.wired.com/2013/09/flux-eyestrain/

138. Tamura, Haruka, Tomoko Nishida, Akio Tsuji, Hisataka Sakakibara. Association Between Excessive Use Of Mobile Phone And Insomnia And Depression Among Japanese Adolescents. Int. J. Environ. Res. Public Health. 2017, 14(7). http://www.mdpi.com/1660-4601/14/7/701/htm

139. WebMD. "Nightime Computer Users May Lose Sleep." June 19, 2003. http://www.webmd.com/sleep-disorders/news/20030620/nighttime-computer-users-may-lose-sleep

140. Jelodar, G, A. Akbari, S. Nazifi. "The prophylactic effect of Vitamin C on oxidative stress indexes in rat eyes following exposure to radiofrequency wave generated by a BTS antenna model. Int J Radiat Biol. 89(2):128-131, 2013.

141. Ober, Clinton, Stephen Sinatra, Martin Zucker. Earthing. Basic Health Publications, Inc. Laguna Beach, California. 2014.

142. Borba, Michele. UnSelfie, Why Empathetic Kids Succeed in Our All-About-Me World. Touchstone Books. New York, New York. 2016. 92.

143. Bounds, K MS; Johnson, A MS; Wolverton, B.C.; NASA Interior Landscape Plants for Indoor Air Pollution Abatement. 1989.

144. United States Environmental Protection Agency. "Household Hazardous Waste Disposal." www.epa.gov/osw/conserve/materials/how.htm.

145. Kalemba, D.; Kunicka, A., Antibacterial and Antifungal Properties of Essential Oils, Current Medicinal Chemistry, Volume 10, Number 10, May 2003, pp. 813-829(17).

146. Martin, D. "5 Toxics that are Everywhere." CNN Health. Toxic America Series. May 2010.

147. Costner, P; Thorpe, B; McPherson,A., "Sick of Dust, Chemicals in Common Household Products". Clean Act Production. March 2005.

148. Mother Teresa. No Greater Love. New World Library. Novato, California. 1989. 129.

149. Terkeurst, Lysa. The Best Yes. Nelson Books. Austin, Texas. 2014.

150. Biello, D. "Plastic (Not) Fantastic: Food Containers Leach a Potentially Harmful Chemical". Scientific American. February 19, 2008.

151. Beth Ann Filiano, Dioxin and Women's Health. Environmental Sciences, Columbia University School of Public Health 3 December 1996.

152. Giglio, Louie. Wired For a Life of Worship. Multnomah Publishers. Sisters, Oregon. 2006. 25-26.

153. Thomas, Gary. Sacred Pathways. Zondervan. Grand Rapids, Michigan. 2010. 50.

154. United States Environmental Protection Agency. "Introduction to Indoor Air Quality". www.epa.gov/iaq/ia-intro.html.

155. Benson, Dr. Herbert. "Toxic Stress Derails Healthy Development". Harvard University Center on the Developing Child.

156. Rodrigo Mendes, Marco Kruijt, Irene de Bruijn, Ester Dekkers, Menno van der Voort, Johannes H. M. Schneider, Yvette M. Piceno, Todd Z. DeSantis, Gary L. Andersen, Peter A. H. M. Bakker, Jos M. Raaijmakers,Deciphering the Rhizosphere Microbiome for Disease-Suppressive Bacteria.*Science* 27 May 2011: Vol. 332, Issue 6033, pp. 1097-1100. DOI: 10.1126/science.1203980.http://science.sciencemag.org/content/332/6033/1097.full

157. Duc Le, Huynh A Hong, Teresa M Barbosa, Simon M Cutting, Characterization of Bacillus Probiotics Available for Human Use. Applied and Environmental Microbiology 70(4):2161-71, May 2004. DOI: 10.1128/AEM.70.4.2161-2171.2004. https://www.researchgate.net/publication/8634403_Characterization_of_Bacillus_Probiotics_Available_for_Human_Use.

158. Woodward, Orrin. Resolved. Obstacles Press. Inc. Flint, Michigan. 2011. 75.

159. Gaarder, Jostein. Sophie's World, A Novel About The History Of Philosophy. Farrar, Straus, and Giroux. New York, New York. 1994. 134.

160. Mercola. Fun Facts About Hugging. February 2014. http://articles.mercola.com/sites/articles/archive/2014/02/06/hugging.aspx.

161. How Porcelain is Made. http://www.madehow.com/Volume-1/Porcelain.html.

About The Author

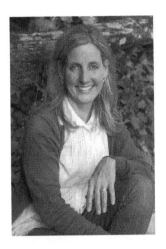

Susan has been teaching, speaking and educating others about well-ness for over 30 years with a focus on mind-body support the past 16 years. She is an experienced registered yoga teacher with 1000+ teaching hours and holds specialty certifications in Thai bodywork, Trauma Sensitive Holy Yoga, Pilates and Aromatherapy. Her personal practice includes caring for her tribe of six kids and serving in youth ministry with her husband . Together they celebrate twenty-five years of marriage. Susan is passionate about supporting teens and women as an advocate for anti-trafficking education, survivor rehabilitation and inspiring life-long changes for her clients. Susan loves to spend time outdoors, hiking and gardening and is courageous to explore new things and enjoys taking on do-it-yourself projects that involve art, restoration, upcycling and bringing out the hidden beauty of her projects. You can follow her living out the healthy, natural lifestyle at www.pureHOMEandBODY.com

www.TwoInchesofWool.com

www.purehomeandbody.com